Disclaimer

The information provided in this skincare book is for general informational purposes only. It is not intended to be a substitute for professional medical advice, diagnosis, or treatment. Always seek the advice of a qualified dermatologist with any questions you may have regarding a medical condition or before adopting any skincare regimen.

Skincare products and practices mentioned in this book may vary in effectiveness and suitability depending on individual circumstances. It is important to consider personal allergies, sensitivities, and skin conditions before incorporating any new skincare products or treatments. Patch testing and consulting with a dermatologist or healthcare professional are recommended to ensure the safety and appropriateness of any skincare regimen. Furthermore, the information in this book is not intended to create a professional-client relationship between the reader and the author or publisher.

The stories mentioned in this book are fictional and intended for illustrative purposes only. Any resemblance to actual persons, living or dead, or actual events is purely coincidental. While the stories are designed to provide relatable examples and engage the reader, they should not be considered real-life experiences or testimonials.

GOOD SKIN
BAD SKIN

Habits that Define your skin

DR. DEEPAK JAKHAR   **DR. ISHMEET KAUR**

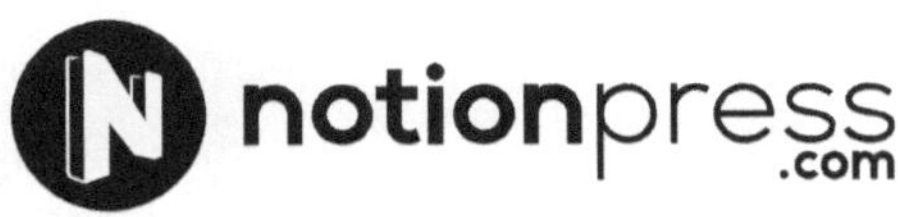

For Evani,

You bring immeasurable joy and laughter into our lives every single day. Your innocent curiosity, natural cuteness, boundless energy, and pure love have enriched our time and made this journey of book writing a joyful one!

Thank you for helping create an amazing cover design

Contents

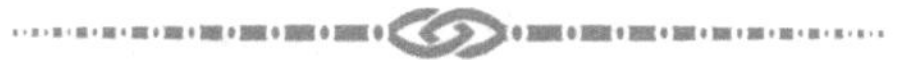

Acknowledgment

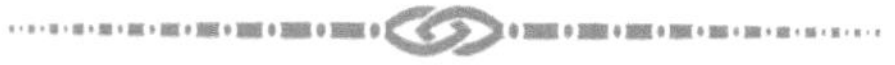

We would like to express our deepest gratitude to our parents, whose unwavering love and support have been a constant source of inspiration throughout this journey. Your encouragement and belief in us have been instrumental in making this book a reality.

To all our family, teachers, and friends, thank you for your continuous encouragement and for being a pillar of strength during the writing process.

We extend our heartfelt appreciation to the team at the publishing house for their guidance, expertise, and dedication in bringing this book to fruition. Your professionalism and support have been invaluable.

Lastly, to the readers, we express our sincere gratitude. It is your curiosity and eagerness to learn that motivate us to share our insights and experiences. We hope that this book will serve as a helpful resource on your journey to discovering the joys and wonders of skincare.

Thank you all for being a part of this incredible adventure!

Why This Book?

Imagine this: You're standing in front of a dazzling array of skincare products, feeling overwhelmed and unsure about which one to choose. Sounds familiar? You're not alone. The world of skincare can be a confusing and daunting place, especially if you don't have a background in dermatology or skincare.

It seems like every brand out there is promising miraculous results, leaving you wondering if they truly deliver or if it's just another marketing ploy. And let's face it, skincare products can be expensive, so wasting your hard-earned money on something that doesn't work is the last thing you want.

It's no secret that the skincare industry is booming, and while there are certainly reputable brands that genuinely care about delivering results, there are also those who are more interested in selling products rather than addressing your skincare concerns. The market is flooded with products boasting a wide range of ingredients, but the truth is, not all of them have been scientifically proven to be effective for your skin. In fact, many lack the rigorous scientific studies needed to back up their claims. Only a select few have been approved by the Food and Drug Administration (FDA), ensuring their safety and efficacy.

To make matters more complicated, there is a lack of knowledge about skincare among the general population. With the rise of social media and influencer culture, it's easy to get swayed by flashy advertisements or popular personalities endorsing certain products. But the truth is, skincare is not a one-size-fits-all solution. What works for someone else may not work for you.

Sure, seeking professional advice from a dermatologist or skincare expert is ideal, but let's be realistic—not everyone has the time or resources to do that for every skincare product they purchase. That's where understanding the basics of skincare becomes crucial.

Based on our extensive experience of meeting and counseling thousands of individuals seeking skincare advice, we've gained valuable insights into their needs and requirements. We've observed that those who have achieved and maintained healthy, glowing skin, share common habits, motivations, and dedication when it comes to skincare.

Our goal is to demystify skincare, providing you with accessible, engaging, and relatable information that empowers you to make informed decisions about your skincare routine. We'll delve into the fundamentals of skincare, helping you understand the science behind it without overwhelming you with technical jargon.

Through this book, we aim to equip you with the knowledge you need to navigate the vast world of skincare products. We'll explore different skin types, common concerns, and the ingredients that have been scientifically proven to be effective. We'll debunk myths, shed light on the marketing tactics used in the industry, and help you separate fact from fiction.

So, whether you're a skincare enthusiast seeking to expand your knowledge or a skincare newbie looking to establish a solid routine, this book is for you. Together, let's embark on a journey to discover the secrets of healthy, radiant skin and empower ourselves to make informed choices for our skincare needs.

SECTION ONE

The Need to Understand Skincare!

SECTION ONE

The Need to Understand Skincare!

Knowledge is the Key

Congratulations if you have decided to read this book and refine your understanding of skincare! The skincare industry is one of the fastest-growing industries in the world and enthusiasm for skincare can be seen among all age groups. Everyone is a part of this skincare revolution. While an abundance of something positive can be delightful, it can also be overwhelming, perplexing, and confusing. The markets are full of skincare products and new products keep coming every day. Ever try to search for any skincare product, like a moisturizer or a sunscreen?

Well, you will come across thousands of brands on the internet, each claiming to be better than the other. Social media platforms are full of influencers and advertisements promoting various skin care regimes, DIY tricks, home remedies, and skincare products. It makes you tempted to try these products by looking at the tall claims made by the various manufacturing and marketing companies. Some products claim to take away the pigmentation in a few weeks, some claim to completely cure acne overnight, others guarantee visible anti-aging benefits with just one application, and so on... But do they actually work?

Let us tell you the story of Ayana. Ms. Ayana visited us one fine day with a bag full of over-the-counter products which she had used over the past two years. She was a salon artist who desperately wanted her skin to look healthy and even-toned. The temptation, she said, was to buy new skincare products and try them on the skin. During this period, she read a lot of skincare blogs/articles, watched social media videos, and believed her favorite influencers. She claimed to spend thousands over the past two years without getting the results she desired. What frustrated her the most was that she couldn't find the reason why nothing was working for her skin. That is the story of many people across the world. Many people who consult for skincare routines these days have already spent quite a lot of time, energy, and money on skincare products and skincare routines. People spend hours researching the products that best suit their skin, yet they end up buying the wrong product. Ever wondered why?

People not only are wasting their time but their hard-earned money on skincare products that might not be beneficial to their skin. With so many products in each category of skincare, people are confused about how to select a product that best suits their skin, without causing any adverse reaction.

The motive of the skincare industry seems to sell products and very few actually care to give results to their customers. The market is flooded with ingredients that have dubious efficacy on the skin. There is very little science behind the efficacy of certain ingredients and scientific studies are lacking to back up their claims. Only a few of them are actually FDA-approved. The situation is worsened by the lack of knowledge about skincare among the general population. The trend is to buy skincare products online after getting influenced by advertisements or influencers. The smart, however, seek professional advice before investing in their products. But, that might not be possible for everyone at all times. Hence arises, the need to understand the basics about skin and its care.

Over the past decade, we have met, discussed, and counseled thousands of individuals seeking skincare advice. During the course of time, we have developed a deep sense of the needs and requirements of these individuals when it comes to skincare. In addition, we have also realized that people who maintain good, healthy skin have some common habits, motivation, and dedication toward skincare.

One of our friends Emma, a woman in her late thirties, has always taken her skincare routine seriously. From a young age, she learned the importance of taking care of her skin and the benefits of investing in high-quality skincare products. As a result, she has developed excellent buying habits when it comes to skincare products.

Emma is a careful and informed shopper. She researches products extensively before making a purchase, reading reviews, and studying the ingredients to ensure that they meet her high standards. She prefers products that use natural, organic, and cruelty-free ingredients and avoid harsh chemicals. Rather than falling for the latest skincare trends or marketing hype, Emma sticks to what works for her skin type and concerns. She knows her skin's needs and chooses products that address specific concerns, such as fine lines and dryness, rather than buying products with unnecessary ingredients or promises.

Emma also values consistency and has a strict skincare routine that she follows religiously. She uses a gentle cleanser, toner, serum, sunscreen and moisturizer every day, as well as a weekly mask or exfoliant. She knows that consistency is key to achieving healthy and glowing skin, and she makes sure to use products consistently to see results.

Another factor that contributes to Emma's good buying habits is her budget-consciousness. While she is willing to invest in high-quality products that work for her skin, she doesn't overspend or fall for high-priced products that don't deliver results. She looks for deals and sales but never sacrifices quality for a bargain. Thanks to her good buying habits and consistent skincare routine, Emma's skin looks youthful, healthy, and radiant. She serves as a role model for others looking to develop healthy skincare habits and reminds us that investing in our skin is an investment in our overall well-being.

Each individual has some specific habits when it comes to skincare and these habits define the outcome their skin achieves. For example, when it comes to buying skincare products, not everyone thinks like Emma. There are some habits that result in bad outcomes. Let's dive into some common habits that people have when buying skincare products, both good and bad.

Good Skin Habits

Research: It's essential to do your homework before selecting a skincare product. Take the time to read reviews, not only about the product itself but also about the key ingredients. For example, if you're considering an XYZ retinol serum, learn about what retinol is, how it affects the skin, and whether it's suitable for your skin type. Look for reviews from users with similar skin concerns to get a better understanding of how the product might work for you.

Read the labels: Always read the list of ingredients of a skincare product. This helps you ensure that the product doesn't contain any ingredients that could potentially irritate your skin. If you have sensitive skin, be cautious of products with fragrances, alcohol, or harsh chemicals.

Consider your skin type: Select a skincare product that is specifically formulated for your skin type. If you have dry skin, look for products that contain moisturizing ingredients like hyaluronic acid or ceramides. Tailoring your products to your skin's needs can help optimize their effectiveness.

Test it out: Before applying a new skincare product all over your face, perform a patch test on a small area of your skin. This helps you check for any allergic reactions or adverse effects. Apply a small amount of the product to the inside of your wrist or behind your ear, and monitor the area for any redness, itching, or irritation for twenty-four hours.

Bad Skin Habits

Impulsive buying: Avoid making impulsive purchases based solely on attractive packaging or marketing claims. Instead, take the time to research the product and its ingredients. This helps you make a more informed decision and increases the chances of finding a product that suits your skin.

Using too many products: It's tempting to try every new skincare product on the market, but using too many products at once can overwhelm your skin. Stick to a simple skincare routine that addresses your specific concerns. This allows your skin to adjust and prevents potential irritation.

Falling for unrealistic promises: Be cautious of products that make unrealistic promises or claim to produce dramatic results overnight. Remember that good skincare takes time and consistency. Be patient with your routine and have realistic expectations for the gradual improvements you'll see over time.

Ignoring expiration dates: Using expired skincare products can be harmful to your skin. Always check the expiration date on the packaging and discard any products that have passed their expiration date. Using expired products can lead to skin irritation, reduced efficacy, or even infection.

By adopting these good habits and avoiding the bad ones, you can make more informed decisions when it comes to choosing skincare products.

Have you ever thought about the habits you have when it comes to buying skincare products? It's an interesting exercise that can kickstart your skincare journey and help you make more informed choices. Let's take a moment to reflect on your own habits and compare them to the ones we'll be discussing in this book.

Throughout this book, we've categorized skincare habits into "good skin habits" and "bad skin habits" based on scientific evidence and our understanding of skincare. By following good habits and being aware of the bad ones, you can make better choices for your skin.

So, let's begin this journey together! In the following sections, we'll delve deeper into these habits, highlighting them and providing insights and advice. Get ready to explore the world of skincare and cultivate habits that will bring you closer to healthier, more radiant skin.

SECTION TWO

....

What is Skin?

SECTION TWO

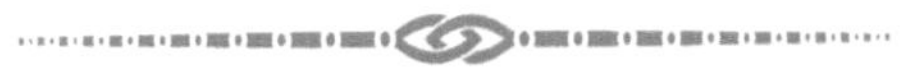

What is Skin?

Unlocking the Secrets of Skin

One of the first things before discussing skincare is to understand the skin itself. Many people, especially untrained influencers, think that they understand skin; but it's a complex organ and it requires years of training to acquire knowledge about skin and how to care for it. We know of a social media influencer who gained a massive following for her beauty and skincare content. She posted pictures and videos of herself using various skincare products and shared her routine with her followers. She claimed to have the perfect solution for every skincare problem, and her followers believed her blindly.

However, what her followers didn't know was that the influencer didn't have any formal education or training in skincare. She relied solely on the information provided by skincare brands and other influencers who also lacked professional knowledge. She often endorsed products that contained harsh ingredients and made false claims about their effectiveness.

Her followers trusted her recommendations and bought the products she promoted, only to end up with damaged skin. Many of them experienced severe reactions, including irritation, redness, and breakouts, and some even had to seek medical attention.

Despite the backlash from her followers, the influencer continued to promote questionable skincare products, ignoring the fact that she was spreading misinformation and causing harm to a lot of people. It wasn't until she faced legal action for false advertising that she realized the gravity of her actions.

We often see people getting influenced by the internet. Samantha, an IT professional, was one such young woman who loved to follow social media influencers for the latest skincare trends and product recommendations. She would spend hours scrolling through Instagram, watching YouTube videos, and reading blog posts about the newest skincare products.

One day, Samantha saw an influencer raving about a new exfoliating scrub that promised to transform her skin. Without doing any research or consulting with a dermatologist, Samantha rushed to purchase the product.

Excited to try her new purchase, Samantha immediately used the scrub that evening. But to her surprise, her skin started to burn and turn red. Panicked, she tried to wash it off, but the damage was already done. She had a severe reaction to the product and her skin was left irritated and inflamed for days.

After this incident, Samantha realized the dangers of blindly following social media influencers when it comes to skincare. She learned the importance of researching ingredients, consulting with a dermatologist, and carefully selecting products that are suitable for her skin type.

Samantha vowed to never let her desire for the latest skincare trends lead her astray from proper skincare practices again. She committed to prioritizing her skin's health and safety above all else and to always doing her due diligence before trying new products.

Why do people keep getting bad skin outcomes? Because they lack the appropriate knowledge about skin. Let's explore the fascinating world of skin and its significance in our overall health. While a comprehensive understanding of the skin would require an entire book, our aim here is to provide you with a brief overview of the scientific facts about skin in an engaging and relatable manner.

Imagine skin as the body's largest organ, covering every inch of our external surface. However, you may have noticed that skin can differ in texture, thickness, and tone across different areas of the body. This is because the skin is composed of three main layers: the epidermis, dermis, and subcutaneous tissue.

Starting with the outermost layer, the epidermis acts as a protective shield against various environmental factors like harmful UV radiation, pollution, and bacteria. It also houses melanocytes, specialized cells responsible for producing melanin, the pigment that gives our skin its unique color.

Beneath the epidermis lies the dermis, which is a crucial layer housing an intricate network of blood vessels, hair follicles, and sweat glands. This layer provides the skin with strength, elasticity, and flexibility. It contains essential proteins like collagen and elastin, which contribute to the skin's structure and resilience.

Deeper still, we find the subcutaneous tissue, the bottommost layer of the skin. This layer consists of fat cells, blood vessels, and nerves. It plays a vital role in regulating body temperature and provides a cushioning effect for our organs and bones.

Now, let's dive into the impressive functions of the skin. Firstly, it serves as a robust barrier, shielding our bodies from external harm. Additionally, the skin helps regulate body temperature, allows us to sense touch and pressure, and even plays a role in synthesizing vitamin

D. It is also involved in immune defense, assisting in wound healing, and maintaining an optimal balance of moisture and oil on the skin's surface.

Considering the significance of skin, it's no wonder that many individuals are motivated to take care of it as part of their overall healthcare routine. Skin is the first thing that catches our attention when meeting someone new, and it often subconsciously influences our perceptions of others. A healthy, glowing, and well-maintained complexion speaks volumes about an individual's self-care habits and can contribute to their confidence in all aspects of life. Such individuals often leave a pleasant impression and radiate a positive energy that attracts others.

The secret behind achieving and maintaining healthy skin is consistency and motivation. Let's explore the different motivations that drive people to embark on their skincare journey. Each person may have their own reasons, and here are some common ones:

a. Improving the appearance of their skin is a top priority for many individuals. They may want to reduce the appearance of acne, wrinkles, fine lines, dark spots, or other skin imperfections. By following a skincare routine tailored to their needs, they hope to achieve a more radiant, even-toned complexion.

b. Maintaining healthy skin is another crucial reason people start caring for their skin. Skincare routines can help keep the skin hydrated, protected from the sun's harmful rays, and shielded from other environmental factors that can damage it. Healthy skin not only looks good but also functions optimally in defending against external aggressors.

c. Addressing specific skin concerns is a common motivation for starting a skincare routine. People with oily skin may want to manage excess oil and shine, while those with dry skin seek products that provide hydration and nourishment. Similarly, individuals with sensitive skin may look for gentle and soothing skincare options, while those with acne-prone skin may focus on products that help manage breakouts.

d. Skincare routines can also serve as a form of self-care and relaxation. The act of caring for one's skin can be a therapeutic experience, providing a sense of pampering and promoting overall well-being. Taking time to nurture and nourish the skin can be a moment of tranquility on a busy day.

e. Preventative measures are another compelling reason to establish a skincare routine. By consistently caring for their skin, individuals can take proactive steps to prevent future skin problems. Regularly protecting the skin from harmful UV rays, maintaining hydration, and incorporating anti-aging ingredients can help ward off premature aging, sun damage, and other skin issues that may arise later in life.

Motivation

Lena had always struggled with maintaining a consistent skincare routine. She would often forget to use the products regularly and gave up after a few weeks. One day, while scrolling through social media, Lena came across a post from us that talked about the benefits of a consistent skincare routine. It explained how regular use of certain products and ingredients can lead to healthier, clearer, and more youthful-looking skin. The post also provided scientific evidence to back up these claims.

For some reason, as she told us later, this post resonated with Lena. She realized that she had never fully understood the rewards behind her skincare efforts. She had only seen skincare as a chore or a trend to follow. But now, she was motivated to change her perspective. Lena decided to research more about skincare and the ingredients that are beneficial for her skin type. With our assistance, she found a few products that contained these ingredients and incorporated them into her daily routine. She also set reminders on her phone to ensure that she used the products at the right times.

After a few weeks, Lena started to notice a difference in her skin. It was clearer, brighter, and more hydrated than before. She was amazed by the results and felt proud of herself for sticking to her routine.

From that day on, Lena understood the rewards of maintaining a consistent skincare routine. She no longer saw it as a challenge but as an investment in her skin's health and appearance. She continued to research and educate herself on skincare, and her skin continued to improve. Lena learned that a little bit of effort and motivation can go a long way in achieving healthy and beautiful skin.

By understanding the benefits of following a proper skincare regimen, you can motivate yourself to make positive changes and embrace a skincare routine that works for you. Let's explore the benefits of following a proper skincare regimen and how it can positively impact your skin and overall well-being.

Protection: Your skin acts as a shield, protecting you from harmful environmental factors like UV radiation, pollutants, and bacteria. Skincare products play a vital role in protecting your skin by forming a barrier, providing antioxidants, and strengthening your skin's natural defenses. By investing in proper skincare, you can enhance your skin's ability to combat these external threats.

Hydration: Dry and dehydrated skin can be more prone to damage, wrinkles, and signs of aging. Skincare products, such as moisturizers, work to replenish and lock in moisture, keeping your skin hydrated and maintaining its moisture balance. Well-hydrated skin appears more plump, supple, and youthful.

Prevention: A consistent skincare routine tailored to your skin type and concerns can help prevent common skin issues. By using appropriate products, you can ward off problems like acne breakouts, hyperpigmentation (dark spots), and premature aging. Prevention is key to maintaining healthy and beautiful skin in the long run.

Treatment: Skincare isn't just about prevention; it can also be effective in treating existing skin issues. With the right products containing active ingredients like salicylic acid (for acne), retinol (for anti-aging), or niacinamide (for inflammation), you can target specific concerns. These ingredients can help reduce inflammation, promote healing, and improve the overall appearance of your skin.

Self-Care: Skincare isn't only about the physical benefits; it's also a form of self-care. Taking the time to pamper your skin and prioritize your personal wellness can have a positive impact on your overall well-being. When you engage in a skincare routine, it becomes a moment of relaxation, self-nurturing, and self-appreciation. This act of self-care can boost your self-confidence, improve your mood, and contribute to a higher quality of life.

Understanding your skin type

Once you have decided to take this journey of skin care, one of the things you need to understand is that every skin is different. Yes, your genetics do play a role in the type of skin you are born with and there is very little you can do to change your skin type. There are several different skin types, each with its own characteristics and specific needs. These skin types are at the core of many of the new-age skincare products. Many products consider it as their USP to be specific for particular skin types. It is very important to understand the different skin types and identify your own. These skin types include:

1. **Normal Skin:** This skin type is balanced, with a healthy complexion and few imperfections. It's not too oily or too dry, and it has a good moisture balance.

2. **Dry Skin:** Dry skin lacks moisture and can appear dull, flaky, or rough. It may feel tight and uncomfortable, especially after washing your face. This type of skin can be more prone to fine lines and wrinkles.

3. **Oily Skin:** Oily skin produces excess sebum, which can make the skin appear shiny or greasy. It may also be prone to clogged pores and acne breakouts.

4. **Combination Skin:** Combination skin has both dry and oily areas, with the T-zone (forehead, nose, and chin) being more prone to oiliness and the cheeks being drier.

5. **Sensitive Skin:** Sensitive skin is easily irritated and may react to certain ingredients or environmental factors. It may appear red, itchy, or inflamed, and can be more prone to allergic reactions and sensitivity to sunlight.

So how do you know what skin type you have? Well, there are a few simple ways:

a. **Wash Your Face:** Start by simply washing your face with a gentle cleanser and patting it dry. Avoid using any skincare products for a few hours before this step. Let it take its natural course.

After your face is clean and dry, wait for thirty minutes and observe your skin in the mirror. Look for any noticeable signs of dryness, oiliness, or a combination of both.

Here are some characteristics to look for

•   **Dry Skin:** If your skin feels tight, flaky, or itchy, and appears dull or ashy, it's likely dry.

- **Oily Skin:** If your skin looks shiny or greasy, especially in the T-zone (forehead, nose, and chin), it's likely oily.

- **Combination Skin:** If your skin is dry in some areas and oily in others, especially in the T-zone, you have combination skin.

- **Normal Skin:** If your skin appears healthy, balanced, and without any noticeable issues, it's likely normal.

- **Sensitive Skin:** If your skin appears easily irritated, red, or inflamed, you may have sensitive skin.

b. **Conduct a Blotting Paper Test:** Another way to determine your skin type is to use blotting paper. Press the blotting paper on different areas of your face, including the T-zone, cheeks, and chin. After a few seconds, remove the paper and observe it.

Here's what to look for

- **Oily Skin:** If the paper has visible oil marks, especially in the T-zone, you have oily skin.

- **Combination Skin:** If the paper shows oil marks only in the T-zone, you have combination skin.

- **Dry Skin:** If the paper doesn't show any oil marks, but your skin feels dry and tight, you have dry skin.

By using these methods, you can determine your skin type and choose skincare products and routines that are appropriate for your skin's specific needs.

Once you have ascertained your skin type, now you would like to focus on various skincare routines. Establishing a daily skincare routine is essential for maintaining healthy and youthful-looking skin. Many people ask us about morning and evening skincare routines.

Let us tell you the various general steps briefly here, the details of individual steps are discussed in subsequent sections.

Morning Skincare Routine

Your morning skincare routine should focus on protecting your skin from environmental stressors and preparing it for the day ahead. Here are the steps to follow for a basic morning skincare routine:

Step 1: Cleanser

Start your day by washing your face with a gentle cleanser to remove any dirt, oil, or impurities that have accumulated on your skin overnight. Use lukewarm water to avoid drying out your skin.

Step 2: Toner

Toning helps to balance your skin's pH levels and prepares it for the next steps in your routine. Choose a toner that is appropriate for your skin type.

Step 3: Serum

Serums are concentrated formulas that deliver active ingredients deep into your skin. Look for a serum that targets your specific skin concerns, such as fine lines, dark spots, or dryness.

Step 4: Eye Cream

The skin around your eyes is delicate and requires special care. Use an eye cream that is formulated to hydrate, brighten, and reduce puffiness and dark circles.

Step 5: Moisturizer

Moisturizing is essential for keeping your skin hydrated and healthy. Choose a moisturizer that is appropriate for your skin type and contains SPF to protect your skin from UV damage. Don't forget your lips.

Step 6: Sunscreen

Apply sunscreen with at least SPF 30 to protect your skin from harmful UV rays. Choose a sunscreen that is broad-spectrum and water-resistant for maximum protection.

Evening Skincare Routine

Your evening skincare routine should focus on repairing and rejuvenating your skin while you sleep. Here are the steps to follow for a basic evening skincare routine:

Step 1: Cleanser

Start by removing any makeup and washing your face with a gentle cleanser to remove dirt, oil, and impurities from your skin.

Step 2: Exfoliant (optional)

Exfoliation helps to remove dead skin cells and stimulate cell turnover. Use a gentle exfoliant once or twice a week to avoid over-exfoliating.

Step 3: Mask (optional)

Masks can help to address specific skin concerns, such as acne, dryness, or dullness. Choose a mask that is appropriate for your skin type and concerns.

Step 4: Toner

Toning helps to balance your skin's pH levels and prepares it for the next steps in your routine. Choose a toner that is appropriate for your skin type.

Step 5: Serum

Use a serum that targets your specific skin concerns, such as fine lines, dark spots, acne or dryness.

Step 6: Eye Cream

Use an eye cream that is formulated to hydrate, brighten, and reduce puffiness and dark circles.

Step 7: Moisturizer

Use a moisturizer that is appropriate for your skin type to keep your skin hydrated and healthy.

By following the steps outlined above, you can create a personalized routine that addresses your specific skin concerns and keeps your skin looking and feeling its best. Remember to choose products that are appropriate for your skin type and always wear sunscreen to protect your skin from UV damage. Whenever in doubt, never hesitate to discuss it with your dermatologist!

SECTION THREE

Basic Skincare

SECTION THREE

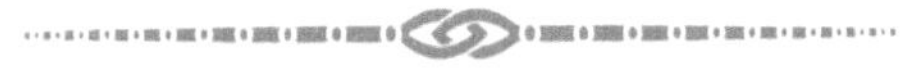

Basic Skincare

Nourish, Protect, Embrace, Repeat!

Some people believe that good skin can only be achieved with high-end skincare regimens. On the contrary, some of the most incredible skincare outcomes are achieved by following the basics of skincare. If the foundation of basic skincare is not there, even the high-end regimens, products, and procedures are useless. The secret to any healthy skin is the consistency of your efforts in skincare. For example, consistency can be in the form of using a good cleanser and sunscreen alone. Indeed, it is better to use these two products consistently for years than to use five different high-end serums for a couple of weeks.

Jane, a theatre artist, had struggled with her skin for years. This affected her social interactions and she would feel under-confident during her performances. She had tried every expensive product on the market, but nothing seemed to work for her. One day, she visited us and on our suggestion decided to simplify her skincare routine and stick to the basics.

She began by washing her face twice a day with a gentle cleanser and followed up with a basic moisturizer. She also started wearing sunscreen every day to protect her skin from the sun's harmful rays. At first, she didn't notice any significant changes in her skin, but she persisted and continued to use the basic skincare routine every day. After a few weeks, she began to notice her skin becoming clearer, smoother, and more radiant.

She was amazed at the difference in her skin's appearance and realized that it was the simple, consistent routine that had made all the difference. She continued to use the basic skincare products and found that her skin looked better than ever before.

Her friends and family noticed the change too and began to ask her what her secret was. Jane happily shared her skincare routine with them, encouraging them to simplify their own routines and stick to the basics. In the end, Jane learned that great skin doesn't necessarily come from using expensive and complicated products. Sometimes, all it takes is a consistent routine with basic skincare products to achieve the beautiful and healthy-looking skin she had always wanted.

Most dermatologists encourage people to stick with the basics of skincare before going for advanced skincare routines. When the basics are strong, you understand the importance of each step of skincare.

Cleansing

This is the first step in any skincare routine. Cleansing involves the use of a gentle cleanser which is used to remove excess oil, dirt, and makeup from the skin. The cleanser should be choosen accroding to the skin type. The basic steps of cleansing typically include the following:

- **Remove Makeup:** The first step in cleansing is to remove any makeup that you may be wearing. This can be done with a makeup remover, micellar water, or cleansing oil.

- **Wet Face:** Once your makeup is removed, wet your face with lukewarm water. It is advisable to avoid hot water for cleaning.

- **Apply Cleanser:** Take a small amount of cleanser and gently massage onto the face in circular motions with the fingertips. Be sure to focus on areas where you tend to have more oil or dirt build-up, such as your T-zone.

- **Rinse:** After you've massaged the cleanser onto your face, rinse it off with lukewarm water. Be sure to rinse thoroughly to ensure that all of the cleanser is removed.

- **Pat Dry:** After rinsing off, use a clean, soft cloth or towel to pat dry the face. Rubbing of the face should be avoided.

Cleansers

When talking about cleansing, we keep coming across the word 'cleanser'. A cleanser is a cosmetic product or preparation used to clean or remove dirt, oil, makeup, and other impurities from the skin. It is typically used on the face, but body cleansers are also available. Cleansers come in various forms, including liquids, gels, creams, foams, and powders, and can be formulated for different skin types.

The purpose of a cleanser is to leave the skin clean, refreshed, and ready for other skincare treatments or makeup applications. Always remember to choose a cleanser that is suitable for your skin type and to be gentle when cleansing your face. Also remember, over cleansing can cause dryness and irritation by stripping the skin of its natural oils. There are several different types of cleansers, each designed to address different skin types and concerns. Most common types of cleansers include:

- **Foaming Cleansers:** Foaming cleansers are usually water-based and create a rich lather when mixed with water. They're great for oily or acne-prone skin because they help to remove excess oil and dirt from the skin. However, they can be drying for people with dry or sensitive skin.

- **Cream Cleansers:** Cream cleansers are thicker and more moisturizing than foaming cleansers, making them great for people with dry or sensitive skin. They're less likely to strip the skin of its natural oils, but may not be as effective at removing heavy makeup or excess oil.

- **Gel Cleansers:** Gel cleansers are usually water-based and have a thicker, gel-like consistency. They're a good option for people with oily or combination skin because they're effective at removing excess oil and impurities without drying out the skin.

- **Oil Cleansers:** Oil cleansers are great for removing heavy makeup and sunscreen, and are gentle enough for all skin types. They work by dissolving oil-based impurities on the skin, leaving it clean and hydrated.

- **Micellar Water:** Micellar water is a gentle, water-based cleanser that uses tiny micelles to attract and remove dirt, oil, and makeup from the skin. It's great for all skin types, but may not be as effective at removing heavy makeup or waterproof products.

Face Washes

Face washes, also known as facial cleansers, are designed to remove dirt, oil, and impurities from the skin. Here are some of the most common types of face washes:

- **Foaming Face Wash:** Foaming face washes are water-based and create a lather when mixed with water. They're great for people with oily or acne-prone skin because they help to remove excess oil and dirt from the skin.

- **Cream Face Wash:** Cream face washes are thicker and more moisturizing than foaming face washes. They're great for people with dry or sensitive skin because they're less likely to strip the skin of its natural oils.

- **Gel Face Wash:** Gel face washes are usually water-based and have a thicker, gel-like consistency. They're great for people with oily or combination skin because they're effective at removing excess oil and impurities without drying out the skin.

- **Exfoliating Face Wash:** Exfoliating face washes contain small particles or acids which removes dead skin cells and unclog pores. They're great for people with acne-prone skin or for those who want to improve the texture and tone of their skin.

- **Oil-Based Face Wash:** Oil-based face washes are great for removing heavy makeup and sunscreen, and are gentle enough for all skin types. They work by dissolving oil-based impurities on the skin, leaving it clean and hydrated.

Soaps

Soap is a common cleaning agent that we use to wash our face, body, and hair. It's made by combining fats or oils with an alkali through a chemical process called saponification. But here's something interesting: Did you know that the pH level of your skin plays a crucial role in maintaining its health?

The skin has a slightly acidic pH level, ranging from 4.5 to 5.5, which helps to protect it and maintain its natural balance. When we use a soap that is too alkaline, it can disrupt this delicate pH balance and cause issues like dryness, irritation, and even breakouts. That's why it's important to choose a soap that is pH balanced to ensure it doesn't harm your skin.

While soaps have been used for centuries, they have been overtaken by cleansers and facewashes in recent times. There are a few reasons for this shift. First, some soaps can be too harsh for the skin, stripping away its natural oils and leaving it dry and irritated. Secondly, certain soaps may contain fragrances or other ingredients that can further irritate sensitive skin.

Moreover, cleansers and facewashes are often formulated specifically for the face, taking into account its unique needs. They effectively remove makeup, dirt, and other impurities without causing harm or disrupting the skin's natural balance. So, if you're looking for a gentle and effective way to cleanse your face, it's usually best to opt for a cleanser or facewash rather than traditional soap.

What is Double Cleansing?

Imagine this, you've had a long day, and it is finally time to unwind and give your skin the care it deserves. You reach for your trusted skincare products, but have you ever wondered if there's more you could be doing to truly cleanse your skin? That's where the concept of double cleansing comes in.

In Asia, where skincare is taken seriously, the pursuit of a flawless complexion is a way of life. It's here that the practice of double cleansing was born. And in recent years, it has gained widespread popularity as people around the world have become captivated by the allure of achieving healthy, glowing skin.

So, what exactly is double cleansing? It's a simple yet effective technique that involves using two different types of cleansers to give your skin a deep and thorough clean. The first cleanser, often an oil-based product, is like a gentle melting potion that effortlessly dissolves makeup, dirt, and excess oil, leaving your skin free from impurities. It's like waving a magic wand over your face, effortlessly removing all traces of the day.

But we're not done just yet. The second cleanser, a water-based product, swoops in to finish the job. Its refreshing touch sweeps away any lingering impurities and ensures your skin is left feeling clean and revitalized. It's like a burst of freshness, washing away the remnants of the day and leaving your skin ready to absorb the goodness that follows.

The benefits of double cleansing are vast and impactful. By incorporating this technique into your skincare routine, you're giving your skin the ultimate cleanse. All the impurities that can clog your pores and lead to breakouts are whisked away, paving the way for a clearer complexion. It's like hitting the reset button, allowing your skin to breathe freely and rejuvenate itself.

But that's not all. Double cleansing also enhances the effectiveness of your other skincare products. By ensuring your skin is thoroughly cleansed, the subsequent products you apply, like serums or moisturizers, are able to penetrate deeper into your skin. It's like creating the perfect canvas for your skincare routine, amplifying the results, and making every drop count.

Now, let's talk about choosing the right cleansers for double cleansing. The options are plentiful, and it's essential to find the ones that suit your skin's unique needs. For the first step, an oil-based cleanser is ideal. Think of it as a gentle melting potion that dissolves makeup effortlessly. Coconut oil, jojoba oil, and argon oil are popular choices that work like magic.

Moving on to the second step, a water-based cleanser is what you need. It can take the form of a foaming cleanser, a gentle cream cleanser, or even the beloved micellar water. The key is to find a cleanser that matches your skin type, as using one that is too harsh can lead to irritation and dryness. It's like finding the perfect partner for your skin, someone who understands and complements its needs.

Ah, there's one more thing to consider—the pH balance. Our skin has a natural pH that is slightly acidic, and using a cleanser that is too alkaline can disrupt its delicate balance. Look for cleansers that are pH balanced or have a pH level close to your skin's natural acidity. It's like maintaining the harmony and integrity of your skin's protective barrier.

While double cleansing is a fantastic technique for many, it's important to remember that it may not be necessary for everyone. If you have dry or sensitive skin, you may find that double cleansing can be too harsh and cause irritation. In such cases, a gentle cleanser that respects your skin's needs might be the better option.

Now that we understand the basics of cleansing, let's take a look at some cleansing habits that can decide your skin outcomes.

Good Skin Habits

- Choosing a cleanser that is appropriate for your skin type and concerns

- Using lukewarm water when cleansing to help open up your pores and remove dirt and impurities

- Being gentle when cleansing, avoiding harsh scrubbing or pulling on the skin

- Rinsing your face thoroughly with water after cleansing to ensure all cleanser and debris are removed

- Following up with a moisturizer to help hydrate and protect the skin

Bad Skin Habits

- Using a cleanser that is too harsh for your skin (this can strip the skin of its natural oils and cause dryness or irritation)

- Using hot water when cleansing (this can further irritate the skin and cause redness or sensitivity)

- Using a cleanser that contains harsh exfoliants like walnut shells or apricot kernels (these can cause micro-tears in the skin)

- Over-cleansing your skin (this can lead to dryness or irritation)

- Using a face wash or cleanser that contains ingredients that you are allergic to

Toning

After cleansing, many people like to use a toner to help remove any remaining dirt or oil from their skin. Toners also help to balance the skin's pH and prepare the skin for the next steps in the routine. In our opinion, use of toner is an add-on step in your skin care. Below are some common types of toners:

- **Hydrating Toners:** Hydrating toners add moisture back into the skin after cleansing. They often contain ingredients like hyaluronic acid, glycerine, or aloe vera to help soothe and hydrate the skin.

- **Exfoliating Toners:** Exfoliating toners contain acids like alpha-hydroxy acids (AHAs) or beta-hydroxy acids (BHAs) that help to exfoliate the skin and unclog pores. They're great for people with acne-prone or dull skin.

- **Clarifying Toners:** Clarifying toners are designed to remove excess oil and impurities from the skin. They often contain ingredients like witch hazel or salicylic acid, which can be drying for some skin types.

- **pH-Balancing Toners:** pH-balancing toners are designed to restore the skin's natural pH level after cleansing. They often contain ingredients like green tea or chamomile extract to soothe and balance the skin.

- **Anti-Aging Toners:** Anti-aging toners often contain antioxidants like vitamin C or retinol, which can help to reduce the appearance of fine lines and wrinkles.

- **Calming Toners:** Calming toners are designed to soothe and hydrate sensitive or irritated skin. They often contain ingredients like chamomile, calendula, or Centella Asiatica extract.

Finding the perfect toner for your skincare routine can seem overwhelming, but fear not! Here are some simple tips to help you choose the right toner for your skin:

1. **Know Your Skin Type:** Is your skin oily, dry, or somewhere in between? Understanding your skin type will help you pick a toner that addresses your specific needs. If you have oily or acne-prone skin, look for toners with ingredients like salicylic acid or witch hazel to keep excess oil at bay. If your skin is dry or sensitive, opt for toners with hydrating ingredients such as hyaluronic acid or aloe vera to replenish moisture.

2. **Consider Your Concerns:** Do you struggle with acne breakouts or want to combat signs of aging? Take your concerns into account when choosing a toner. Choose toners that contain exfoliating ingredients like AHAs or BHAs if you're prone to breakouts. For anti-aging benefits, seek out toners with antioxidants like vitamin C or retinol to help reduce fine lines and wrinkles.

3. **Check Those Ingredients:** Take a closer look at the ingredients list on the toner bottle. Look for ingredients that are beneficial for your specific skin type and concerns. Avoid toners that contain alcohol or fragrance, as these can be harsh and irritating for some skin types.

4. **Give It a Test Run:** Before fully committing to a new toner, it's a good idea to test it out first. Try a sample or perform a patch test on a small area of your skin to make sure it doesn't cause any adverse reactions or breakouts. Better safe than sorry!

5. **Follow the Instructions:** Each toner may have its own set of instructions for application. Be sure to read and follow the directions provided on the label or consult with a dermatologist if needed. Some toners are designed for once-daily use, while others can be used twice a day. Consistency is key!

Remember, when applying toner, be gentle and avoid rubbing or scrubbing your skin too harshly. You can use a cotton pad or your clean hands to lightly pat or press the toner onto your skin. Treat your skin with care, and it will thank you!

Now that we understand the basics about toners, let's take a look at some toner habits that can decide your skin outcomes.

Good Skin Habits

- Choosing a toner that is appropriate for your skin type and concerns

- Using a toner after cleansing to help balance the skin's pH and remove any remaining impurities

- Applying toner with a cotton pad or your fingertips, gently patting it onto your skin

- Looking for toners with hydrating ingredients like hyaluronic acid or aloe vera to help soothe and moisturize the skin

- Incorporating toner into your skincare routine as needed, based on your skin's individual needs

Bad Skin habits

- Using toner that contains alcohol (this can be drying and irritating for some skin types)

- Overusing toner (this can lead to dryness or irritation)

- Using toner as a replacement for cleansing (it is not meant to remove makeup or dirt from the skin)

- Applying toner too aggressively or scrubbing your skin with the cotton pad (this can cause irritation)

- Using toner that contains ingredients that you are allergic to or have had a negative reaction to in the past

Moisturization

The next step in a basic skincare routine is moisturizing, which involves applying a moisturizer to your skin to help keep it hydrated and nourished. Many people suffer from dry and irritated skin and moisturiser can be their best friend. But it is important to choose the right one. Let us tell you the story of Sophie.

Sophie, a social activist, had always struggled with her skin. She had tried everything (fancy creams and lotions) to get rid of the dry patches and the occasional breakouts, but nothing seemed to work. She had given up hope and had just accepted that her skin was always going to be problematic. That was until she discovered the power of a proper moisturizer.

Referred to us by a common friend, we noticed her struggling with her skin. After a thorough skin examination, she was recommended a moisturizer that contained ingredients specifically designed to hydrate her dry skin. Sophie was skeptical, to begin with, but she decided to give it a try after we counseled her. She went home and started using the moisturizer as instructed. After just a few days, she noticed a difference. Her skin was smoother and more hydrated than it had been in years. The dry patches that had plagued her for so long were gone.

As Sophie continued to use the moisturizer, she noticed that her skin was becoming more radiant. People started commenting on how healthy she looked, and she even started to get compliments on her skin. She couldn't believe that something as simple as a moisturizer had made such a difference. Sophie had always been self-conscious about her skin, but now she felt confident and beautiful. She even started experimenting with makeup, something she had always avoided because she didn't like the way it looked on her skin.

Sophie's journey with her new moisturizer has been life-changing. It has given her the confidence to try new things and to feel good about herself. Sophie now knows that her skin isn't perfect, but it is much better than it had ever been before.

Moisturization is a science and it's important to choose a moisturizer that is appropriate for your skin type. There are several different types of moisturizers, each formulated to meet the unique needs of different skin types and concerns. Here are some of the most common types of moisturizers:

1. Creams

Creams are thick and emollient, making them an excellent choice for those with dry or mature skin. They provide deep hydration and help to nourish and protect the skin.

2. Lotions

Lotions are lighter than creams and are typically water-based. They are ideal for those with normal to oily skin and are easily absorbed into the skin, providing hydration without feeling heavy or greasy.

3. Gel Moisturizers

Gel moisturizers are lightweight and typically water-based, making them a great choice for those with oily or acne-prone skin. They absorb quickly and help to hydrate the skin without clogging pores.

4. Facial Oils

Facial oils are typically made from natural plant oils and are great for those with dry or mature skin. They help to nourish and hydrate the skin, providing a healthy glow and improving the appearance of fine lines and wrinkles.

5. Serums

Serums are lightweight and designed to penetrate deeply into the skin, delivering potent ingredients like vitamins, antioxidants, and hyaluronic acid. They are a great choice for those with specific skin concerns like anti-aging, hyperpigmentation, or acne.

Now that you have an idea of the different types of moisturizers available, it's time to learn about the essential steps for effective moisturization. These steps will help you make the most of your moisturizer and ensure your skin stays hydrated and healthy. So, let's dive in!

General Steps to Apply Moisturizer

1. **Start with a Clean Face:** Wash your face with a gentle cleanser and pat dry with a clean towel. This helps to remove any dirt, oil, or makeup that may be on your skin. The use of a toner after cleansing is optional.

2. **Take an Appropriate Amount of Moisturizer:** Squeeze or pump out a small amount of moisturizer onto your fingertips or palm. The amount of moisturizer you need may vary based on your skin type and the specific product you're using.

3. **Apply the Moisturizer:** Using your fingertips, gently massage the moisturizer onto your face and neck in upward circular motions. Be sure to cover your entire face, including your forehead, cheeks, nose, and chin, and don't forget to apply moisturizer to your neck as well.

4. **Don't Forget Your Eye Area:** If you're using a separate eye cream, apply it gently with your finger around your eyes, Try not to pull or tug on the sensitive skin around your eyes.

5. **Let It Absorb:** Allow the moisturizer to absorb into your skin for a few minutes before applying any makeup or sunscreen. This helps to ensure that the moisturizer is fully absorbed into your skin, providing maximum benefits.

6. **Apply as Needed:** You may need to apply moisturizer multiple times throughout the day, depending on your skin's needs and the climate you are in. It's important to listen to your skin and adjust your moisturizing routine as needed.

Overall, the key is to be gentle when applying moisturizer, using upward circular motions to help stimulate blood flow and promote healthy, glowing skin.

Moisturizer for Atopic Skin

Atopic dermatitis, commonly known as eczema, is a skin condition that affects millions of people worldwide. It can cause dry, itchy, and inflamed skin that can be challenging to manage. One of the essential steps in managing atopic skin is moisturization. Moisturizers help to hydrate and soothe the skin, reducing the severity of symptoms.

Why Moisturization is Vital for Atopic Skin?

The skin acts as a protective barrier against external factors such as pollution, sun exposure, and microorganisms. In people with atopic skin, this barrier function is compromised, making the skin more susceptible to irritants and allergens. Moisturizers help to replenish the skin's moisture content, strengthening its barrier function and reducing the risk of flare-ups.

Atopic skin is also characterized by a deficiency in skin lipids such as ceramides. Ceramides play a crucial role in maintaining the skin's barrier function, preventing water loss, and protecting against environmental stressors. A moisturizer that contains ceramides can help to restore the skin's lipid balance and improve its overall health.

Types of Moisturizers for Atopic Skin

When choosing a moisturizer for atopic skin, it is essential to select one that is gentle, non-irritating, and fragrance-free. Look for moisturizers that contain emollients (petrolatum, mineral oil, and dimethicone), humectants (glycerine, hyaluronic acid, and urea), and ceramides. Ceramides are a type of lipid that helps to maintain the skin's barrier function. They form a protective layer on the skin's surface, preventing water loss and protecting against environmental stressors.

Tips for Moisturizing Atopic Skin

Atopic skin can be quite demanding, but with a little extra care, you can keep it happy and healthy. Let's dive into some tips for moisturizing atopic skin that will leave you feeling nourished and comfortable. First, make moisturizing a regular habit throughout the day, especially after bathing or showering. Remember, lukewarm water is your friend! Avoid the temptation of hot water, which can strip away precious oils. Instead, gently pat your skin dry with a soft towel, treating it like the delicate treasure it is. And here's a pro tip: when applying your moisturizer, strike while the iron is hot—or, in this case, while your skin is still slightly damp—to lock in that much-needed moisture. Oh, and be selective with your skincare products! Steer clear of harsh soaps, fragrances, and alcohol, opting for gentle, hypoallergenic options instead.

To keep your skin feeling fresh and breezy, choose loose-fitting, breathable clothing made from natural fibers like cotton. And for an extra boost of moisture, consider bringing a humidifier into your home, infusing the air with soothing hydration. Remember, your atopic skin deserves some tender love and care, so embrace these tips and watch your skin flourish with happiness.

Now that we understand the importance of moisturization, let's take a look at some moisturization habits that can decide your skin outcomes.

Good Skin Habits

- Choosing the right moisturizer for your skin type: Different skin types require different types of moisturizers. Choose a moisturizer that is appropriate for your skin type and concerns.

- Applying moisturizer to clean skin: Always apply moisturizer to clean skin to ensure maximum absorption and effectiveness.

- Using a gentle touch: Use gentle, upward circular motions to apply moisturizer, and be careful not to rub or pull on your skin.

- Being consistent: Use a moisturizer daily, and adjust the frequency based on your skin's needs.

- Layering appropriately: If you're using multiple skincare products, apply moisturizer after toner and serum but before sunscreen.

Bad Skin Habits

- Using too much moisturizer: Using too much moisturizer can clog pores and make your skin feel greasy. Using a pea-sized amount for your entire face is sufficient in most individuals.

- Applying moisturizer to dirty skin: Applying moisturizer to skin that is not clean can cause breakouts and prevent the moisturizer from being absorbed properly.

- Skipping sunscreen: Moisturizer can help hydrate your skin, but it doesn't provide enough protection from the sun. Always use a separate sunscreen on top of your moisturizer.

- Using expired products: Expired moisturizers can lose their effectiveness and potentially cause skin irritation.

—   Assuming one moisturizer fits all: Not all moisturizers work for everyone, and it's essential to find the one that works best for your skin type and concerns

Sunscreen

Rachel, a young enthusiastic woman, loved spending time outdoors on the weekends and soaking up the sun, whether it was at the beach, the park, or on a hike in the mountains. Rachel had always heard about the importance of wearing sunscreen to protect her skin from the harmful rays of the sun, but she never really took it seriously.

One summer day, Rachel went to the beach for a vacation with her friends. She brought a towel, a book, and a bottle of water, but she forgot to bring sunscreen. Rachel didn't think it was a big deal, and she thought that the sun wouldn't be too strong that day. So she lay down on the sand and started reading her book.

As the day went on, Rachel started to feel the heat of the sun on her skin. She could feel her skin starting to burn, but she didn't want to leave the beach yet. She thought she could tough it out and stay in the sun a little longer.

After a few more hours, Rachel's skin had turned bright red and was extremely painful to the touch. She knew she had made a mistake by not wearing sunscreen. The next few days were some of the worst of Rachel's life. Her skin was incredibly sensitive, and it hurt to wear clothes or even touch the affected areas. Rachel couldn't sleep properly because of the pain, and she had to miss work because she couldn't concentrate.

Rachel eventually came to see us, and we told her that she had suffered from a severe sunburn. Rachel was shocked to learn this, and she realized that she had been taking her skin's health for granted. From that day on, Rachel always made sure to wear sunscreen when she went outside. She now knows that it was an essential part of protecting her skin from the sun's harmful rays. Rachel learned that prevention was better than cure, and she didn't want to risk getting another painful sunburn or worse, developing skin cancer.

Ready for a sunscreen adventure? Let's explore the wonderful world of sun protection! Sunscreen is not just a cosmetic product; it's a crucial tool for protecting our skin from the harmful effects of the sun. Just like superheroes shield us from harm, sunscreen swoops in to protect our skin from the sun's powerful rays. Wearing sunscreen can prevent painful sunburns, premature aging, reduce the risk of skin cancer, and help us maintain healthy skin for years to come. Wearing sunscreen is an essential step in any skincare routine. But did you know there are different types of sunscreen to save the day? Let's uncover the secrets!

First up, we have physical sunscreen! With ingredients like zinc oxide and titanium dioxide, it creates an invisible shield on your skin, reflecting those harmful UV rays away. Perfect for the sensitive souls out there, it's gentle yet effective in guarding your precious skin.

Now, meet the chemical sunscreen! It's like a secret agent, working undercover to absorb those sneaky UV rays and transform them into harmless heat. Since it's lightweight, it absorbs completely into the skin, making it a go-to for everyday protection.

But wait, how do you choose the perfect sunscreen for your skin? First, look for sunscreen with a Sun Protection Factor (SPF) of 30 or higher. This magical number shields your skin from those pesky sunburns. But we're not done yet! Ensure your sunscreen offers broad-spectrum protection, guarding against both UVB and UVA rays. It's like having a double superhero team on your side!

Now, let's dive into sunscreen for different skin types. Dry skin in need of some hydration? Seek out sunscreen with ingredients like glycerine or hyaluronic acid, quenching your skin's thirst while protecting it from the sun's fury. Is oily skin feeling left out? Fear not! Look for oil-free formulas that won't add to the shine, letting you enjoy sun-kissed adventures without greasy aftermath.

Sensitive skin, we've got your back too! Find a sunscreen specially designed for your delicate skin, free from fragrances, and packed with gentle ingredients like zinc oxide or titanium dioxide. And for our acne-prone friends, opt for oil-free or non-comedogenic sunscreens that won't clog your pores. Stay clear and protected with lightweight, gel-based formulas that won't leave you feeling like you've slathered on a goopy mask.

It's important to keep in mind that everyone's skin is unique, and what works for one person may not work for another. It's always a good idea to do a patch test before trying a new sunscreen. At the same time, it is important to know the pros and cons of different sunscreen formulations, such as lotion, spray, and gel-based sunscreens, so that you can choose the most suitable option for your needs. Below we will discuss the pros and cons of various formulations of sunscreen.

Lotion Sunscreen

Pros:

— Moisturizing: Lotion sunscreens often contain moisturizing ingredients, which can be beneficial for those with dry or sensitive skin.

— Even coverage: Lotion sunscreens can be easier to apply and provide more even coverage than spray or powder sunscreens.

— Versatile: Lotion sunscreens can be used on both the face and body.

 — Convenient packaging: Many lotion sunscreens come in convenient packaging, such as a squeeze tube or pump bottle, which makes them easy to apply and travel with.

Cons:

 — Greasy or heavy: Some lotion sunscreens can feel greasy or heavy on the skin, which may not be ideal for those with oily or acne-prone skin.

 — Takes time to absorb: Lotion sunscreens can take a few minutes to absorb into the skin, which may not be ideal if you are in a hurry.

 — May leave a white cast: Some lotion sunscreens contain physical blockers like zinc oxide or titanium dioxide, which can leave a white cast on the skin, especially on darker skin tones.

 — May cause breakouts: Some lotion sunscreens can clog pores and cause breakouts, especially if they contain comedogenic ingredients like fragrances or oils.

Overall, lotion sunscreens can be a good option for those looking for a versatile and moisturizing sunscreen. However, it's important to choose a lotion sunscreen that is appropriate for your skin type and concerns and to reapply sunscreen every two hours or more often if you are swimming or sweating.

Cream-Based Sunscreen

Pros:

 — Moisturizing: Cream-based sunscreens often contain moisturizing ingredients, which can be beneficial for those with dry or sensitive skin.

- Longer lasting: Cream-based sunscreens are often more resistant to water and sweat than other types of sunscreens, making them a good option for outdoor activities.

- Versatile: Cream-based sunscreens can be used on both the face and body.

- Suitable for sensitive skin: Cream-based sunscreens are often formulated to be gentle and non-irritating, making them a good option for those with sensitive skin.

Cons:

- May be greasy: Some cream-based sunscreens can feel greasy or heavy on the skin, which may not be ideal for those with oily or acne-prone skin.

- Takes time to absorb: Cream-based sunscreens can take a few minutes to absorb into the skin, which may not be ideal if you are in a hurry.

- May leave a white cast: Some cream-based sunscreens contain physical blockers like zinc oxide or titanium dioxide, which can leave a white cast on the skin, especially on darker skin tones.

- May cause breakouts: Some cream-based sunscreens can clog pores and cause breakouts, especially if they contain comedogenic ingredients like fragrances or oils.

Overall, cream-based sunscreens can be a good option for those looking for a longer-lasting and moisturizing sunscreen.

Gel Sunscreen

Pros:

- Lightweight: Gel sunscreens are typically lighter in texture and feel than cream or lotion sunscreens, making them a good option for those with oily or acne-prone skin.

- Absorbs quickly: Gel sunscreens are often formulated to absorb quickly into the skin, which can be convenient if you're in a hurry or don't want to wait for your sunscreen to dry.

- Non-greasy: Because gel sunscreens are lightweight and fast-absorbing, they are less likely to leave a greasy or heavy feeling on the skin.

- Non-comedogenic: Gel sunscreens are often non-comedogenic, meaning they are less likely to clog pores and cause breakouts.

Cons:

- May not be moisturizing enough: Because gel sunscreens are lightweight, they may not be moisturizing enough for those with dry or dehydrated skin.

- Limited options: Gel sunscreens are not as widely available as cream or lotion sunscreens, so it may be more difficult to find one that meets your specific needs.

- May not be water-resistant: Gel sunscreens may not be as water-resistant as other types of sunscreens, which may be a concern if you plan on swimming or sweating.

- May contain alcohol: Some gel sunscreens contain alcohol, which can be drying and irritating to the skin.

Overall, gel sunscreens can be a good option for those looking for a lightweight, non-greasy sunscreen that absorbs quickly.

Spray Sunscreen

Pros:

- Easy to apply: Spray sunscreens are convenient to use on hard-to-reach areas like the back or shoulders.

- Fast-drying: Spray sunscreens typically dry quickly, which can be convenient if you're in a hurry.

- Lightweight: Spray sunscreens are often lightweight and non-greasy, making them a good option for those with oily or acne-prone skin.

- Water-resistant: Spray sunscreens are often water-resistant, which can be convenient if you plan on swimming or sweating.

Cons:

- Uneven application: Spray sunscreens can be difficult to apply evenly, which may lead to missed spots or patches of skin that are not fully protected.

- Inhalation risk: There is a risk of inhaling spray sunscreen particles, which can be harmful if inhaled in large amounts over time.

- Limited coverage: Spray sunscreens can be difficult to control and may not provide as much coverage as cream or lotion sunscreens.

- Potential for skin irritation: Some spray sunscreens contain alcohol or other ingredients that can be drying or irritating to the skin.

Overall, spray sunscreens can be a convenient and quick option for sunscreen application, especially for hard-to-reach areas. However, it's important to use caution when applying spray sunscreen to avoid inhalation and ensure even coverage.

Brand Value of a Sunscreen

Often we see people who have already purchased sunscreen based on their internet search, friend suggestion, or dermatologist recommendation. With so many brands around, sometimes investing in sunscreen with a brand value makes more sense. Brand value is an important factor, as it can give you an idea of the quality, reliability, and effectiveness of the product. A sunscreen brand with a strong reputation and positive reviews from customers is likely to be more trustworthy than a brand that is less well-known or has a history of negative feedback.

By choosing a sunscreen brand with a strong brand value, you can be more confident that the product will provide the sun protection that you need and that it will be safe to use. Additionally, well-known sunscreen brands often have a long history of research and development, which can lead to products that are more innovative and effective.

How to Read the Label of a Sunscreen?

Reading the label of a sunscreen is important because it allows you to understand the ingredients and characteristics of the product, which can help you choose a sunscreen that is effective and safe for your skin. Sunscreens come in different formulations, with varying levels of sun protection, ingredients, and properties. By reading the label, you can determine whether a sunscreen is suitable for your skin type, provides the level of sun protection you need, and meets your personal preferences and needs. Additionally, reading the label can help you identify potential allergens or irritants in the sunscreen, such as fragrances or certain types of preservatives, which can trigger an allergic reaction or cause skin irritation. By knowing what ingredients to look for and avoid, you can minimize the risk of adverse reactions and select a sunscreen that is safe and effective for you. The various terms used on the labels of a sunscreen include:

- **Sun Protection Factor (SPF):** The SPF indicates the level of protection the sunscreen provides against UVB radiation, which is the type of radiation that causes sunburn. The higher the SPF number, the more protection the sunscreen provides.

It is recommended to use a sunscreen with an SPF of 30 or higher.

- **PA Factor:** It is a measure of a sunscreen's protection against UVA radiation, which can penetrate deeper into the skin and cause long-term damage, such as premature aging and skin cancer. PA stands for "protection grade of UVA" and is a system commonly used in Asia to measure UVA protection. PA ratings range from PA+ to PA++++, with higher ratings indicating greater protection against UVA radiation. A sunscreen with a PA+ rating provides some protection against UVA radiation, while a sunscreen with a PA++++ rating provides the highest level of protection against UVA radiation.

- **Broad Spectrum:** Choose a sunscreen which protects against both, UVA and UVB radiations. UVA radiation can cause premature aging and skin damage, while UVB radiation causes sunburn.

- **Water Resistance:** If you plan to be in the water or sweating, invest in a for a water-resistant sunscreen. The label will indicate how long the sunscreen will remain effective in water.

- **Noncomedogenic:** This term means that the sunscreen is formulated to not clog pores or cause acne breakouts. If you have acne-prone skin, look for a sunscreen that is labeled as noncomedogenic.

- **Fragrance-Free:** Some sunscreens contain added fragrances, which can irritate sensitive skin. If you have sensitive skin, look for a fragrance-free sunscreen.

- **Oil-Free:** If you have oily or acne-prone skin, look for a sunscreen that is labeled as oil-free.

- **Allergen-Free:** Some sunscreens are formulated to be free of common allergens, such as nuts or gluten. If you have allergies, look for a sunscreen that is labeled as allergen-free.

- **Active Ingredients:** Check the list of active ingredients to ensure that they are effective in providing sun protection. The most common active ingredients in sunscreens include titanium dioxide, zinc oxide, avobenzone, octinoxate, etc.

- **Skin Sensitivity:** If you have sensitive skin, look for a sunscreen that is formulated for sensitive skin or is labeled as hypoallergenic.

- **Expiration Date:** Sunscreens have a shelf life of about three years, so check the expiration date to ensure that the sunscreen is still effective.

Once you have finalized a sunscreen, you should know the amount of sunscreen to be used for achieving adequate protection. Many people know that they have to apply sunscreen, thanks to the internet and social media aggressive campaigns, but they are not aware of the correct steps of its application. Here are the general steps to apply sunscreen:

1. **Choose the Right Sunscreen:** Look for a broad-spectrum sunscreen that offers protection against both UVA and UVB rays, and has a minimum SPF of 30.

2. **Apply Enough Sunscreen:** Always apply a uniform and generous amount of sunscreen. A good rule of thumb is to use about one ounce (or a shot glass full) of sunscreen to cover your entire body. The magic number to remember for the face is a nickel-sized amount, about a teaspoon.

3. **Apply Sunscreen Before Going Outside:** Apply sunscreen fifteen to thirty minutes before sun exposure to give it time to absorb into the skin.

4. **Apply Sunscreen Evenly:** An even application of sunscreen is essential to provide adequate photoprotection. For the face, start by squeezing that teaspoon-sized amount of sunscreen

onto your fingertips. Then, dot it on your forehead, cheeks, nose, and chin. Spread it gently making sure to reach every nook and cranny, including the often-neglected areas like your ears and the delicate skin around your eyes.

5. **Reapply Sunscreen Regularly:** Reapply sunscreen every two-three hours, or more often if you are swimming or sweating.

6. **Don't Forget Your Lips:** Use a lip balm with SPF to protect your lips from the sun.

7. **Use Sunscreen Every Day:** Even on cloudy or overcast days, UV rays can still penetrate the skin, so it's important to use sunscreen every day.

Remember, using sunscreen is an important step in protecting your skin from the damaging effects of the sun. By following these steps, you can help ensure that your skin is well-protected and healthy. At last, your habits towards the application of sunscreen makes all the difference in the protection offered by it.

Good Skin Habits

- Choosing a sunscreen with an SPF of at least 30, and preferably 50 or higher

- Applying sunscreen generously to all exposed skin, including your face, ears, neck, and any other areas not covered by clothing

- Reapplying sunscreen every two hours or after swimming, sweating, or towel-drying.

- Applying sunscreen at least fifty minutes before sun exposure to give it time to absorb into your skin

- Using sunscreen even on cloudy days, as UV rays can still penetrate through clouds.

- Using a water-resistant sunscreen if you will be swimming or sweating

- Wearing protective clothing, such as a wide-brimmed hat and long-sleeved shirt, in addition to using sunscreen

Bad Skin Habits

- Relying on sunscreen alone to protect you from the sun's harmful UV rays (Seek shade whenever possible and avoid the sun during peak hours of ten a.m. to four p.m.)

- Using expired sunscreen or sunscreen that has been exposed to high temperatures or sunlight.

- Skimping on sunscreen or use too little (be generous with your application and reapply regularly)

- Forgetting to protect your lips with a lip balm that contains sunscreen.

Sunscreen for Children

As parents, we want to do everything we can to protect our children, including their delicate skin. A sunscreen is an essential tool in the fight against harmful UV rays, but with so many options available, it can be hard to know where to start. Children have sensitive skin that is more prone to sunburns and long-term damage from UV rays. Sunburns in childhood can increase the risk of skin cancer later in life. That's why it's important to start protecting your child's skin early on with a high-quality sunscreen.

Choosing the Right Sunscreen for Children

When choosing a sunscreen for children, look for one that is specifically designed for kids. These sunscreens are usually labeled with "child" or "baby" and are formulated with gentle, non-irritating ingredients. Avoid sunscreens that contain fragrances, preservatives, or other harsh chemicals that can irritate your child's skin. Look for a sunscreen with an SPF of at least 30. Water-resistant sunscreens are also a good choice if your child will be swimming or sweating.

How to Apply Sunscreen to Children?

- Start by applying sunscreen to your child's face, ears, neck, and any other exposed areas of skin.

- Use enough sunscreen to form a thick, even layer. For children, a good rule of thumb is to use about one ounce of sunscreen per application.

- Rub the sunscreen in gently, making sure to cover all areas of the skin.

- Reapply sunscreen every two hours or after swimming, sweating, or toweling off.

- Encourage your child to wear protective clothing, such as hats and long-sleeved shirts, to further protect their skin from the sun's harmful rays.

With this information, we believe that now you know the basic aspects of skincare and skincare products. We now move towards advanced skincare in the next section.

SECTION FOUR

Advance Skincare

SECTION FOUR

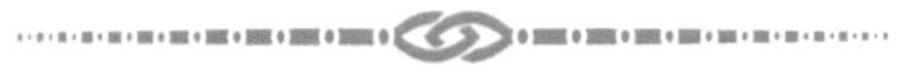

Advance Skincare

There was a middle-aged entrepreneur named Emily. She was a hard-working individual who always kept herself busy with her job, hobbies, and friends. However, Emily had always neglected her skin, thinking that she didn't need to pay too much attention to it. As time passed, Emily started to notice small wrinkles forming around her eyes and mouth. She also noticed that her skin was becoming dull and rough. She tried to cover it up with makeup, but it only made things worse. Emily felt embarrassed and self-conscious about her appearance, which started to affect her confidence.

One day, Emily met an old friend whom she hadn't seen in years. Emily was shocked to see how young and radiant her friend looked, despite being older than her. Emily asked her friend what her secret was, and her friend told her about the importance of advanced skincare. Emily's friend explained that as we age, taking care of your skin isn't just about applying moisturizer and sunscreen. It's about investing in good-quality skincare products that target specific skin concerns, such as fine lines, wrinkles, and dullness. She recommended that Emily try an advanced skincare routine after consulting with us.

Emily was hesitant at first, thinking that it would be too expensive and time-consuming. However, she realized that investing in her skin was worth it. She visited us and discussed her skin concerns. We made a skincare routine best suited for her skin needs.

Within a few weeks, Emily started to notice a significant difference in her skin's texture and appearance. Her wrinkles had reduced, and her skin looked brighter and smoother. Emily felt more confident and happier, knowing that she was taking care of herself. As Emily continued her skincare routine, she also started to notice that her skin was becoming healthier and more resilient. She didn't get as many breakouts or irritations, and her skin felt more hydrated and supple.

At last, Emily learned the importance of advance skincare and how it can positively impact your self-esteem and overall well-being. Taking care of your skin isn't just a luxury; it's a necessity that everyone should invest in. Emily was grateful for her friend's advice and looked forward to maintaining her skincare routine for years to come.

Let us give you several reasons to switch to an advanced skincare routine once you are well-versed in basic skin care:

Healthy Skin

Advanced skin care can help to promote healthy skin by addressing a variety of skin concerns, such as acne, aging, hyperpigmentation, and dryness. By using the right products and techniques, you can improve the appearance and health of your skin.

Prevention

Advanced skin care can also help to prevent future skin problems. For example, using sunscreen daily can prevent sun damage and reduce the risk of skin cancer.

Self-Care

Taking care of your skin can be an act of self-care, helping you to feel more confident and improve your overall well-being.

Anti-Aging

Advanced skin care techniques and products can also help to reduce the signs of aging, such as fine lines and wrinkles.

Personalization

Advanced skin care allows you to personalize your routine based on your skin type, concerns, and lifestyle factors. By tailoring your skin care routine to your individual needs, you can achieve better results and avoid using products that may not be effective for your skin.

An advanced skincare routine is a comprehensive approach to skincare that involves multiple steps (including basic skincare) and advanced techniques to promote healthy, glowing skin. While the specifics of an advanced skincare routine can vary depending on individual skin concerns and needs, some key elements may include:

- **Cleansing:** An advanced skincare routine typically includes a double cleansing process to thoroughly remove dirt, oil, and makeup from the skin.

- **Exfoliation:** Advanced skincare routines may include gentle physical or chemical exfoliation to remove dead skin cells and promote cell turnover.

- **Targeted Treatments:** Advanced skincare routines may involve the use of targeted treatments such as serums, ampoules, or facial oils to address specific skin concerns such as fine lines, wrinkles, hyperpigmentation, or acne.

- **Moisturizing:** An advanced skincare routine typically includes a hydrating moisturizer to nourish and protect the skin.

- **Sun Protection:** Daily sun protection is crucial to an advanced skincare routine to prevent premature aging and reduce the risk of skin cancer. A broad-spectrum sunscreen with an SPF of 30 or higher should be applied daily, even on cloudy days.

- **Facial Massage and Tools:** An advanced skincare routine may include facial massage or tools such as gua sha or jade rollers to promote lymphatic drainage, improve circulation, and enhance product absorption.

- **Customization:** An advanced skincare routine is customized to an individual's skin type, concerns, and lifestyle factors, allowing for a personalized approach to skincare.

Overall, an advanced skincare routine involves a comprehensive approach to skincare that prioritizes the health and appearance of the skin through a combination of targeted treatments, hydrating and nourishing products, and sun protection.

Exfoliation

Ram was a middle-aged, physically fit successful entrepreneur but his skin was dull, uneven, and prone to breakouts, and he often felt self-conscious about his appearance. At his friend's suggestion, he decided to visit us to see if there was anything he could do to improve his skin. After carefully examining his skin, we suggested that he try exfoliation, which involves removing the outer layer of dead skin cells to reveal the fresher, brighter skin underneath.

Ram had heard that exfoliation could be harsh on the skin. But we assured him that there were gentle methods that would not damage his skin. We recommended that Ram use a chemical exfoliant, as these would be less abrasive than physical exfoliants like scrubs.

Ram decided to give it a try and began incorporating exfoliation into his skincare routine. At first, he didn't notice much of a difference, but after a few weeks, he began to see a noticeable change in his skin. His complexion was brighter and more even, and his pores appeared smaller. He also noticed that his breakouts were less frequent and his skin looked smoother and more hydrated. Ram was amazed at the transformation that exfoliation had brought about in his skin's appearance.

Over time, he continued to use exfoliation as a regular part of his skincare routine and saw even more improvements in his skin. His confidence grew, and he no longer felt self-conscious about his skin's appearance.

Sometimes the simplest solutions can make the biggest difference. Only a few know that gentle exfoliation can be a crucial part of maintaining healthy, radiant skin. By taking the time to exfoliate regularly, one can transform the skin in greater ways.

Exfoliation is the process of removing dead skin cells from the surface of the skin. Dead skin cells can build up on the skin's surface, making it appear dull, dry, and rough. By removing these dead skin cells, exfoliation can help to improve the texture and appearance of the skin, while also allowing for better product absorption.

There are two main types of exfoliation: physical and chemical.

Physical Exfoliation

Physical exfoliation involves physically scrubbing the skin with a textured product or tool, such as a scrub, brush, or sponge. This can be an effective way to remove dead skin cells, but it's important to use gentle pressure and avoid over-exfoliating, which can cause irritation and damage to the skin.

Chemical Exfoliation

Chemical exfoliation involves the use of alpha-hydroxy acids (AHAs) or beta-hydroxy acids (BHAs) to dissolve the bonds between dead skin cells and the skin's surface, allowing them to be easily removed. Chemical exfoliants can be milder than physical exfoliants and are generally better suited for sensitive or acne-prone skin. Alpha-hydroxy acids (AHAs) include glycolic acid, lactic acid, and mandelic acid, while beta-hydroxy acids (BHAs) include chemicals like salicylic acid. Besides AHA and BHA, chemical exfoliation includes the use of fruit enzymes such as papaya, pineapple, or pumpkin enzymes; polyhydroxy acids (PHAs) such as gluconolactone and lactobionic acid and retinoids such as retinol and tretinoin.

Manual Exfoliation

Manual exfoliation involves using a tool, such as a microdermabrasion device or a dermaplaning tool, to manually remove dead skin cells from the skin's surface. This is done by an expert dermatologist and should not be performed at home.

Exfoliation can be done one or two times a week, depending on skin type and sensitivity. It's important to let your dermatologist choose the frequency of exfoliation to avoid over-exfoliating, which can cause redness, dryness, and irritation.

Serums

Serums are lightweight, highly concentrated skincare products that are formulated to deliver a potent dose of active ingredients to the skin. Unlike moisturizers, which are designed to hydrate and protect the skin, serums are typically formulated to address specific skin concerns, such as fine lines, wrinkles, hyperpigmentation, or acne.

Serums can contain a variety of active ingredients, depending on their intended purpose. Some common active ingredients in serums include:

- **Vitamin C:** An antioxidant that can help to brighten the skin and reduce the appearance of dark spots and hyperpigmentation.

- **Hyaluronic Acid:** A humectant that can help to hydrate and plump the skin.

- **Retinol:** A derivative of vitamin A that can help to reduce the appearance of fine lines and wrinkles and improve skin texture.

- **Niacinamide:** A form of vitamin B3 that can help to reduce the appearance of pores and improve skin texture.

- **Peptides:** Short chains of amino acids that can help to stimulate collagen production and improve skin elasticity.

Serums are typically applied after cleansing and toning the skin but before moisturizer. They are designed to penetrate deeply into the skin to deliver active ingredients where they are needed most. Because they are highly concentrated, a little bit of serum goes a long way.

It's important to choose a serum that is appropriate for your skin type and specific skin concerns.

Scottie was excited to try a new face serum that her friend had recommended. The packaging looked attractive, and the product claimed to work wonders on her skin type. Without a second thought, she applied a generous amount of the serum to her face and neck. The next morning, Scottie woke up to a nightmare. Her face had broken out into a severe rash with red bumps, and her skin felt tight and itchy.

Distressed, Scottie visited us, and we diagnosed her with an allergic reaction to the face serum. We explained that patch testing was a crucial step in determining if a skincare product was suitable for an individual's skin type. Had Scottie done a patch test, she could have avoided the unpleasant reaction.

From that day on, Scottie realized the importance of patch-testing new skincare products. She learned that just because a product works well for someone else, it doesn't mean it would work well for her. She understood that patch testing would give her skin a chance to react to the product in a controlled environment and would allow her to identify any potential side effects before using it.

Scottie shared her story with her friends and family and advised them always to do a patch test before using any new skincare product. She realized that taking a few minutes to patch test could save a lot of time, money, and discomfort in the long run.

Patch Test

Patch testing is a crucial step in introducing new skincare products into your routine. It can help prevent adverse reactions, minimize skin irritation, and ensure that the product is suitable for your skin type. By taking the time to patch test, you can save yourself from a lot of unnecessary discomfort and ensure that your skin stays healthy and glowing. Here are the steps to do a patch test at home:

- Choose a small, inconspicuous area on your skin, such as the inside of your wrist or behind your ear.

- Cleanse the area with a gentle cleanser and pat it dry.

- Apply a small amount of the skincare product to the area and wait for it to dry.

- Leave the product on for at least twenty-four hours, and during this time, avoid getting the area wet or applying any other skincare products to it.

- If you experience any itching, burning, redness, or swelling during the twenty-four-hour period, remove the product immediately and rinse the area with cool water.

- If you do not experience any adverse reactions during the twenty-four-hour period, you can assume that the product is safe for use. Remember, in some cases, the reactions can develop up to forty-eight hours after application.

How to Choose a Vitamin C Serum?

Vitamin C serums have gained popularity due to their ability to improve the overall health and appearance of the skin. The anti-aging benefits, brightening effect, protection from environmental stressors, versatility, and ease of use make vitamin C serums a popular choice for many people. Vitamin C is a potent antioxidant that fights free radical damage, promotes collagen synthesis, reduces the appearance of dark spots and hyperpigmentation, and protects against UV rays and pollution. Additionally, vitamin C serums can be used by people of all skin types and ages, making them a highly sought-after skincare product.

When choosing a vitamin C serum, there are a few factors to consider:

Type of Vitamin C

There are different types of vitamin C available in the market, such as ascorbic acid, ascorbyl palmitate, and tetrahexyldecyl ascorbate. Ascorbic acid is the most potent form of vitamin C, but it can be unstable and prone to oxidation. Ascorbyl palmitate and tetrahexyldecyl ascorbate are more stable but may be less effective. Consider your skin type and concerns and choose a vitamin C serum that contains the form of vitamin C that is most suitable for your skin.

Concentration of Vitamin C

Look for a vitamin C serum with a concentration of ten to twenty percent, which has been shown to be effective in improving skin texture, brightening skin tone, and reducing the appearance of fine lines and wrinkles. Higher concentrations can irritate the skin, especially for sensitive skin types.

pH Level

Vitamin C is most effective at a pH level between three and 4.5. Look for a vitamin C serum with a pH within this range to ensure optimal absorption and effectiveness.

Additional Ingredients

Look for a vitamin C serum that contains additional ingredients that can enhance its benefits, such as vitamin E, ferulic acid, hyaluronic acid, and niacinamide. These ingredients can help to improve skin hydration, protect against free radical damage, and enhance the brightening effects of vitamin C.

Packaging

Vitamin C is prone to oxidation and can lose its effectiveness when exposed to light, air, and heat. Look for a vitamin C serum that is packaged in an opaque, airtight container to protect it from degradation.

One important thing to consider before buying any serum is that nothing works uniformly for all skin types. You should always study the side effect profile of any skincare product before buying. There was a young woman named Ilina who had heard a lot about the benefits of vitamin C serum for the skin from her friend. Excited to try it out for herself, she purchased a bottle of the serum and started using it daily. At first, Ilina was pleased with the results. Her skin looked brighter and more even-toned, and she received compliments from friends and family. However, after a few weeks of use, Ilina started experiencing some side effects. Her skin had become dry and flaky, and she noticed some redness and irritation on her cheeks. She also experienced some breakouts, which was unusual for her as she had never had acne before.

Concerned about these side effects, she did some research and discovered that vitamin C serums can sometimes cause skin irritation and sensitivity, especially if used in high concentrations or by people with sensitive skin.

Disappointed with the side effects, she stopped using the serum and switched to a gentler skincare routine. She learned that while vitamin C serums can be beneficial for some people, they are not suitable for everyone and can have side effects if used incorrectly. From then on, Ilina made sure to research and carefully consider any skincare products before incorporating them into her routine, and she was grateful for the lesson she learned from her experience with the side effects of vitamin C serum.

Here are some habits when it comes to choosing and using a vitamin C serum:

Good Skin Habits

- Patch testing: Before using Vitamin C serum for the first time, patch test it on a small area of skin to make sure you don't have any allergic reaction.

- Applying to clean skin: Make sure your skin is clean and dry before applying vitamin C serum to help it penetrate better.

- Using sunscreen: Vitamin C can make your skin more sensitive to the sun, so make sure to use sunscreen during the day.

- Storing properly: Vitamin C serum can oxidize and become less effective if exposed to light and air, so store it in a cool, dark place and make sure the bottle is tightly closed after use.

— Following instructions: Follow the instructions on the packaging for how much to use and how often to apply.

Bad Skin Habits

— Mixing with other active ingredients: Avoid mixing vitamin C serum with other active ingredients, such as retinol or AHAs/BHAs, as they can reduce its effectiveness.

— Applying too much: Using too much vitamin C serum can irritate your skin, so start with a small amount and gradually increase if needed.

— Using on broken skin: Avoid using vitamin C serum on broken or irritated skin, as it can cause further irritation.

— Expecting overnight results: Vitamin C serum takes time to work, so be patient and consistent with your use to see results.

— Using the expired product: Make sure to check the expiration date of your vitamin C serum and discard it if it has expired.

How to Choose a Retinol?

Retinoids are a class of compounds derived from vitamin A that are commonly used in skincare products and prescription medications for their ability to improve the appearance of the skin and treat certain skin conditions. Retinoids work by stimulating cell turnover, promoting collagen production, and reducing the production of sebum (oil) in the skin. Some common retinoids include:

- **Retinol:** This is the most commonly used over-the-counter retinoid in skincare products.

- **Retinaldehyde:** This is a less common over-the-counter retinoid that is gentler than retinol.

- **Adapalene:** This is a prescription-strength retinoid that is used to treat acne.

- **Tretinoin:** This is a prescription-strength retinoid that is used to treat acne and reduce the appearance of fine lines and wrinkles.

- **Isotretinoin:** This is a prescription-strength retinoid that is used to treat severe acne.

Retinoids can be very effective, but they can also cause skin irritation and sensitivity, so it is important to use them as directed and under the guidance of a healthcare professional.

Retinol is a popular anti-aging ingredient that can help improve the appearance of fine lines, wrinkles, and uneven skin tone. Here are some factors to consider when choosing a retinol serum:

- **Strength:** Retinol comes in different strengths, ranging from 0.001% to 1%. If you're new to using retinol, start with a lower-strength product and work your way up to avoid skin irritation.

- **Formulation:** Retinol serums come in different formulations, such as creams, gels, and oils. Choose a formulation that suits your skin type and preferences.

- **Other Ingredients:** Look for a retinol serum that contains other beneficial ingredients, such as antioxidants, hyaluronic acid, etc., which can help enhance the effectiveness of the retinol and provide additional benefits for your skin.

- **Brand Reputation:** Choose a retinol serum from a reputable brand that uses high-quality ingredients and has positive customer reviews.

- **Packaging:** Retinol can break down when exposed to air and light, so choose a serum that comes in opaque packaging or has airless pump technology to protect the product's potency.

- **Price:** Retinol serums can range in price from affordable to expensive. Consider your budget when choosing a product, but keep in mind that high-quality retinol serums can be an investment in your skin's health and appearance.

Many people nowadays use retinol in their skin care routines, without consulting a dermatologist. Whereas this approach might work for some, and save some extra money (which you might have given as consultation to your dermatologist), it is not a good idea to choose a retinol by yourself. Consulting your dermatologist and discussing your skincare needs might help you choose a better retinol product.

John was a middle-aged YouTuber with thousands of followers. He talked about new technology in the mobile industry on his channel. He was concerned about the appearance of fine lines and wrinkles on his face. Some of his followers who have followed him for years started commenting about his age on his channel and this made him very uncomfortable. He had heard about the benefits of using retinol in skincare products and decided to start using an over-the-counter retinol cream without consulting with a dermatologist first.

At first, John was pleased with the results. He noticed that his skin appeared smoother and more radiant. However, after a few weeks, he started experiencing redness, flakiness, and irritation on his face. He thought that this might be a normal side effect of using retinol, so he continued to use the product.

As time passed, John's skin became increasingly sensitive and inflamed. He began to develop acne-like bumps on his face, and his skin felt painful and itchy. He became worried and thus decided to visit us. We examined John's skin and diagnosed him with a condition called retinoid dermatitis, which is a type of skin irritation caused by retinoids. John was advised to stop using the retinol cream immediately.

John learned his lesson the hard way that it is important to consult with a dermatologist before using retinol products. While retinoids can be very effective in improving the appearance of the skin, they can also cause serious skin irritation and other side effects if not used properly.

Here is a checklist of habits for using retinol:

Good Skin Habits

- Patch testing: Before using retinol serum for the first time, patch test it on a small area of skin to make sure you don't have any allergic reaction.

- Starting slowly: If you're new to retinol, start with a low concentration and gradually increase the frequency and amount over time to avoid irritation.

- Applying at night: Retinol can increase the sensitivity of your skin to sun, so it's best to apply it at night and use sunscreen during the day.

- Moisturization: Retinol can be drying, so make sure to apply a moisturizer after using it to help hydrate your skin.

- Being patient: Retinol takes time to work, so be patient and consistent with your use to see results.

Bad Skin Habits

- Using with other active ingredients: Avoid using retinol with other active ingredients, such as AHAs/BHAs or vitamin C, as they can reduce its effectiveness or cause irritation.

- Applying too much: Using too much retinol can cause irritation, so start with a small amount and gradually increase if needed.

- Using on broken skin: Avoid using retinol on broken or irritated skin, as it can cause further irritation.

- Using during pregnancy: Retinol is not recommended for use during pregnancy or breastfeeding.

- Using the expired product: Make sure to check the expiration date of your retinol serum and discard it if it has expired.

Can You Use Retinol and Vitamin C Together?

Yes, retinol and vitamin C can be used together in a skincare routine, but it's important to use them correctly to avoid any potential irritation or adverse reactions.

When using both retinol and vitamin C together, it's recommended to apply them at different times of the day to prevent potential irritation. Vitamin C is best used in the morning, as it can help to protect against environmental stressors and boost the effectiveness of sunscreen. Retinol is best used at night, as it can increase skin sensitivity to sunlight and may cause irritation when used with vitamin C.

It's also important to start with a low concentration of retinol and vitamin C and gradually increase over time to avoid overwhelming the skin. Additionally, it's important to use a moisturizer to help soothe and hydrate the skin, as both retinol and vitamin C can be drying. If you have sensitive skin or are concerned about using both retinol and vitamin C together, it's best to consult a dermatologist for personalized advice.

How to Choose Niacinamide?

Niacinamide, also known as vitamin B3 or nicotinamide, is a water-soluble vitamin that is commonly found in foods such as meat, fish, and leafy vegetables. It is also consumed as a dietary supplement and is used in skincare products for its many benefits for the skin.

Niacinamide is a very versatile ingredient in skincare products, and it has been shown to have many different benefits for the skin, including:

- **Improving the Skin's Barrier Function:** Niacinamide helps to strengthen the skin's barrier, which can help to reduce moisture loss and protect the skin from environmental stressors.

- **Reducing Inflammation:** Niacinamide has anti-inflammatory properties, which can help to reduce redness and irritation in the skin.

- **Decreasing the Appearance of Pores:** Niacinamide can help to reduce the size of pores and improve the overall texture of the skin.

- **Reducing Hyperpigmentation:** Niacinamide has been shown to help reduce the appearance of dark spots and hyperpigmentation on the skin.

- **Boosting Collagen Production:** Niacinamide can help to stimulate the production of collagen in the skin, which can help to improve skin firmness and reduce the appearance of fine lines and wrinkles.

Niacinamide is a popular skincare ingredient these days and when choosing a niacinamide product, you should consider the following factors:

- **Concentration:** Look for a product that contains at least five percent niacinamide. Higher concentrations can provide even more benefits, but it's important to start with a lower concentration if you're new to using niacinamide.

- **Formula:** Niacinamide can be found in a variety of skincare products, including serums, moisturizers, and toners. Choose a formula that works best for your skin type and concerns.

- **Other Ingredients:** Look for a product that contains other beneficial ingredients, such as antioxidants, hyaluronic acid, or ceramides. These ingredients can help to enhance the benefits of niacinamide and provide additional skincare benefits.

- **Brand Reputation:** Try to choose a brand that has a good track record, uses high quality ingredients and produces effective skincare products.

- **Other Preferences:** Consider your personal preferences, such as fragrance-free, cruelty-free, or vegan products.

When considering Niacinamide, do keep in mind these habits:

Good Skin Habits

- Patch testing: Before using niacinamide serum for the first time, patch test it on a small area of skin to make sure you don't have any allergic reaction.

- Applying to clean skin: Make sure your skin is clean and dry before applying niacinamide serum to help it penetrate better.

- Using sunscreen: Niacinamide doesn't make your skin more sensitive to the sun, but it's always a good idea to use sunscreen during the day to protect your skin.

- Using with other active ingredients: Niacinamide can be used with other active ingredients, such as vitamin C or retinol, to provide additional benefits for your skin.

- Following instructions: Follow the instructions on the packaging for how much to use and how often to apply.

Bad Skin Habits

- Using with acidic products: Avoid using niacinamide with highly acidic products, as they can reduce its effectiveness.

- Applying too much: Using too much niacinamide serum can cause irritation, so start with a small amount and gradually increase if needed.

- Using on broken skin: Avoid using niacinamide serum on broken or irritated skin, as it can cause further irritation.

- Expecting overnight results: Niacinamide takes time to work, so be patient and consistent with your use to see results.

- Using the expired product: Make sure to check the expiration date of your niacinamide serum and discard it if it has expired.

How to Choose Alpha hydroxy acids (AHAs)?

Alpha hydroxy acids (AHAs) are a group of water-soluble acids that are commonly used in skincare products for their ability to exfoliate the skin and improve its texture and appearance. AHAs are derived from fruit and milk sugars, and they dissolve the bonds between dead skin cells, allowing them to be sloughed away more easily.

There are several types of AHAs, including glycolic acid, lactic acid, citric acid, malic acid, and tartaric acid. Each of these acids has a slightly different molecular size and properties, which can affect their effectiveness and suitability for different skin types.

Some of the benefits of using AHAs in skincare products include:

1. **Exfoliating the Skin:** AHAs improve the skin texture by removing the dead skin cells and promoting the cell turnover.

2. **Smoothing Rough, Dry Skin:** AHAs can help to soften and smooth rough, dry patches of skin, leaving it feeling soft and hydrated.

3. **Reducing Hyperpigmentation:** AHAs can help to reduce the appearance of dark spots and hyperpigmentation on the skin, giving it a more even tone.

4. **Minimizing the Appearance of Pores:** AHAs can help to unclog pores and reduce their size, making the skin appear smoother and more refined.

AHAs such as glycolic acid and lactic acid are used to exfoliate the skin, helping to remove dead skin cells and improve its texture and tone. When choosing AHAs for your skincare routine, there are a few things to consider to help you find the best one for your skin:

- **Skin Type:** AHAs can be beneficial for all skin types, but some AHAs may be better suited for certain skin types. For example, glycolic acid is typically recommended for normal to oily skin, while lactic acid is better for dry or sensitive skin.

- **Concentration:** AHAs come in different concentrations, ranging from five percent to thirty percent or higher. Always start with a lower concentration, and then gradually increase the concentration as per your skin tolerance.

- **pH Level:** AHAs work best at a pH level of three to four, so look for products with a pH within this range to ensure maximum effectiveness.

- **Formulation:** Consider the formulation (cleansers, toners, serums, and masks) that best fits your skincare routine and personal preferences.

- **Other Skincare Products:** If you're using other active ingredients like retinoids or benzoyl peroxide, be cautious about adding AHAs to your routine, as they can cause irritation when combined.

- **Patch Test:** As with any new skincare product, it's important to patch test AHAs on a small area of skin to make sure you don't have an allergic reaction or experience irritation.

How to Choose Beta Hydroxy Acid (BHA)?

Beta hydroxy acids (BHAs) Beta hydroxy acids (BHAs) are a class of chemical compounds that are commonly used in skincare products. The most common BHA used in skincare is salicylic acid, which is derived from willow bark. BHAs are oil-soluble, which means they are able to penetrate deeply into the pores to exfoliate dead skin cells and help unclog pores.

BHAs are known for their ability to treat acne, as well as other skin concerns such as blackheads, whiteheads, and uneven skin texture. They are also effective at reducing the appearance of fine lines and wrinkles and can help improve the overall tone and texture of the skin.

When choosing a BHA for your skincare routine, here are some things to consider:

- **Skin Type:** BHAs are typically recommended for those with oily or acne-prone skin, as they can help to unclog pores and reduce breakouts. However, they can also be used by those with other skin types.

- **Concentration:** BHAs come in different concentrations, ranging from 0.5% to two percent. If you're new to BHAs, start with a lower concentration and gradually increase as your skin tolerates it.

- **pH Level:** BHAs work best at a pH level of three to four, so look for products with a pH within this range to ensure maximum effectiveness.

- **Formulation:** BHAs can be found in a variety of skincare products, including cleansers, toners, serums, and masks. Consider the formulation that best fits your skincare routine and personal preferences.

- **Other Skincare Products:** If you're using other active ingredients like retinoids or AHAs, be cautious about adding BHAs to your routine, as they can cause irritation when combined.

- **Active Ingredient:** The most common BHA is salicylic acid, but other options like betaine salicylate or willow bark extract may be suitable for those with sensitive skin or those who are allergic to salicylic acid.

- **Patch Test:** As with any new skincare product, it's important to patch test BHAs on a small area of skin to make sure you don't have an allergic reaction or experience irritation.

Polyhydroxy Acids (PHAs)

Polyhydroxy acids (PHAs) are a group of chemical exfoliants that are similar to alpha-hydroxy acids (AHAs) and beta-hydroxy acids (BHAs). PHAs are larger molecules that have multiple hydroxyl groups, making them more gentle and less irritating on the skin than AHAs and BHAs. PHAs work by breaking down the bonds between dead skin cells on the surface of the skin, allowing them to be easily removed and revealing smoother, brighter, and more even-toned skin underneath. PHAs are also known to provide hydration to the skin and improve its barrier function. Some common types of PHAs include gluconolactone, lactobionic acid, and maltobionic acid.

How to Choose Between AHA, BHA or PHA?

Your dermatologist would be the best guide to help you choose between the AHA, BHA and PHA. As a general guide, it's important to consider your skin type and concerns when it comes to choosing between polyhydroxy acids (PHAs), alpha hydroxy acids (AHAs), and beta hydroxy acids (BHAs).

PHA is a gentle exfoliant that is suitable for all skin types, including sensitive skin. It can help improve skin texture, brighten skin tone, and reduce the appearance of fine lines and wrinkles. It is also known for its hydrating properties, which can help improve skin's moisture levels.

AHAs are typically used to treat signs of aging, such as fine lines, wrinkles, and age spots. They can also help improve skin texture and tone, as well as promote skin cell turnover. However, AHAs can be more irritating to the skin, particularly for those with sensitive skin.

BHAs are best suited for those with oily or acne-prone skin. They can help unclog pores and reduce the appearance of blemishes. BHAs can penetrate deep into the pores, and since they are oil soluble, can remove excess oil and debris.

Let us see some skin habits when it comes to AHAs, BHAs and PHAs:

Good Skin Habits

- Starting slow: If you're new to using AHAs or BHAs, start with a lower concentration and gradually increase as your skin adjusts.

- Wearing sunscreen: AHAs and BHAs can increase skin sensitivity to the sun, so it's important to wear sunscreen daily to protect your skin.

- Following instructions: Follow the instructions on the product label carefully to ensure you use the product correctly.

- Applying to clean skin: Apply AHAs and BHAs to clean, dry skin for optimal results.

- Using at the right time: AHAs and BHAs are best used in the evening as they can make skin more sensitive to sunlight.

- Moisturization: After applying AHAs and BHAs, it's important to hydrate the skin with a moisturizer.

Bad Skin Habits

- Overusing: Overusing AHAs and BHAs can cause irritation and sensitivity. Start slowly and gradually increase the frequency of use as your skin adjusts.

- Using with other exfoliants: Avoid using AHAs and BHAs with other exfoliants, such as scrubs or brushes, as it can lead to over-exfoliation and irritation.

- Using on broken skin: Avoid using AHAs and BHAs on broken or irritated skin as it can cause further damage and irritation.

- Using with retinol: Avoid using AHAs and BHAs with retinol or other active ingredients that can cause sensitivity and irritation.

- Applying to eye area: Avoid applying AHAs and BHAs to the eye area as it can be too harsh for the delicate skin around the eyes.

- Applying on lips: Avoid applying AHAs and BHAs to the lips as it can cause irritation and dryness.

Peptides

Peptides are short chains of amino acids that act as building blocks of proteins. Peptides when used as active ingredients, can help to improve firmness, fine lines and wrinkles.

Peptides work by signaling the skin to produce more collagen, elastin, and other proteins that contribute to the structure and elasticity of the skin. When applied topically, peptides can penetrate the skin and stimulate these processes, leading to firmer, smoother, and more youthful-looking skin.

Skincare products can have various different peptides, each with a specific function. For example, some peptides work to improve the overall texture and tone of the skin, while others are specifically designed to target fine lines and wrinkles. Some peptides can even help brighten and even out skin tone.

It's also important to pay attention to the concentration of peptides in a product, as well as the overall formulation. Some peptides may be more effective when combined with other ingredients, like antioxidants or hyaluronic acid, so look for products that have a well-rounded formula.

Overall, peptides can be a beneficial addition to a skincare routine for those looking to improve the signs of aging or overall skin health. By understanding the specific benefits of different types of peptides and selecting products with well-formulated ingredients, you can choose a peptide-based skincare product that works best for your unique skin concerns.

Here are some of the most common types of peptides used in skincare products:

- **Palmitoyl Tripeptide-1 (Pal-GHK):** This peptide is often used to help improve skin elasticity and reduce the appearance of fine lines and wrinkles.

- **Palmitoyl Tetrapeptide-7 (Pal-KTTKS):** This peptide helps to reduce inflammation in the skin and can also help to improve the appearance of dark circles under the eyes.

- **Acetyl Hexapeptide-8:** Also known as Argireline, this peptide is often used in anti-aging products to help reduce the appearance of wrinkles by inhibiting muscle contractions.

- **Copper Peptides:** Copper peptides are a type of peptide that contains copper, which has been shown to have anti-inflammatory and antioxidant properties. Copper peptides can help to improve skin texture and firmness, and may also help to reduce the appearance of fine lines and wrinkles.

- **Matrixyl:** This peptide is often used in anti-aging products to help stimulate collagen production, which can help to improve skin texture and reduce the appearance of fine lines and wrinkles.

- **Hexapeptide-9:** This peptide is often used in skincare products to help improve hydration and reduce the appearance of fine lines and wrinkles.

How to Choose Peptides for Your Skin Care?

When choosing a peptide serum, consider the following factors to help you find the best one for your skin:

- **Skin Type:** Peptide serums can benefit all skin types, but some peptides may be better suited for certain skin types. For example, copper peptides may be better for those with dry or mature skin, while Argireline may be better for those with oily or acne-prone skin.

- **Skin Concerns:** Peptides can address a variety of skin concerns, including fine lines and wrinkles, dullness, and uneven texture. Consider the specific skin concerns you want to address and look for a peptide serum that targets those concerns.

- **Concentration:** Peptide serums come in different concentrations, ranging from 1% to 10% or higher. If you're new to peptide serums, start with a lower concentration and gradually increase as your skin tolerates it.

- **Formulation:** Peptide serums can be found in a variety of formulations, including water-based, oil-based, and gel-based. Consider the formulation that best fits your skincare routine and personal preferences.

- **Other Skincare Products:** If you're using other active ingredients like retinoids or AHAs, be cautious about adding a peptide serum to your routine, as they can cause irritation when combined.

- **Active Ingredients:** Look for a peptide serum that contains the specific peptides that have been shown to be effective for your skin concerns.

- **Patch Test:** As with any new skincare product, it's important to patch-test peptide serums on a small area of skin to make sure you don't have an allergic reaction or experience irritation.

Face Masks

In the world of skincare, face masks have become the ultimate self-care treat and a powerful tool in advanced skincare routines. From nourishing to exfoliating to hydrating, there is a face mask for every skin concern. Below we'll dive into the fascinating world of face masks and explore how they can elevate your skincare game, leaving you with radiant and glowing skin.

The Purpose of Face Masks

Face masks are like an easily accessible goodness for your skin. They help in delivering targeted ingredients deep into the skin, providing intensive nourishment and addressing specific concerns. Whether you're looking to hydrate, detoxify, brighten, or tighten your skin, there's a face mask tailored to your needs.

Types of Face Masks

1. **Hydrating Masks:** These masks replenish moisture and restore hydration levels, perfect for dry or dehydrated skin.

2. **Clay or Mud Masks:** Known for their purifying properties, these masks help draw out impurities and excess oil, making them ideal for oily or acne-prone skin.

3. **Exfoliating Masks:** These masks gently slough away dead skin cells, promoting a smoother and more radiant complexion.

4. **Sheet Masks:** Infused with serums, sheet masks provide a quick and convenient way to deliver active ingredients and give your skin an instant boost.

5. **Gel Masks:** With their cooling and soothing properties, gel masks are fantastic for calming sensitive or irritated skin.

The Benefits of Incorporating Face Masks

1. **Deep Cleansing:** Face masks help remove deep-seated dirt, oil, and impurities that regular cleansing may miss.

2. **Enhanced Hydration:** Masks infuse the skin with moisture, providing intense hydration and plumping up the skin.

3. **Improved Skin Texture:** Exfoliating masks help refine the skin's texture, leaving it smoother, softer, and more even-toned.

4. **Targeted Treatment:** Face masks can address specific concerns like acne, fine lines, dullness, or hyperpigmentation, helping to improve the overall appearance of the skin.

5. **Relaxation and Self-Care:** Applying a face mask is a pampering experience that allows you to unwind, destress, and indulge in a little self-care. It's a wonderful way to take a break from the hustle and bustle of daily life.

How to Incorporate Face Masks into Your Skincare Routine?

a. **Cleanse and Exfoliate: Start** with a clean canvas by cleansing your face thoroughly. Exfoliating beforehand can further enhance the benefits of the mask.

b. **Apply the Mask:** Follow the instructions on the product and apply an even layer of the mask to your face, avoiding the delicate eye and lip areas.

c. **Relax and Enjoy:** Take this opportunity to relax, close your eyes, and let the mask work its magic. Listen to calming music, read a book, or simply enjoy a moment of tranquility.

d. **Rinse and Moisturize:** Rinse off the mask with water after the recommended time. Follow up with your favorite moisturizer to lock in hydration.

Face masks are more than just a skincare trend; they are a powerful tool for achieving healthy and radiant skin. By incorporating face masks into your skincare routine, you can address specific concerns, boost hydration, and indulge in some well-deserved self-care. So, grab your favorite face mask, put your feet up, and let the magic unfold, revealing a glowing complexion that will leave you feeling confident and beautiful.

SECTION FIVE

Common Skincare Concerns

SECTION FIVE

Common Skincare Concerns

Troubles to Triumph

In today's world, with social media and constant exposure to images of "perfect" skin, it's easy to feel self-conscious about your own skin. But the truth is, nearly everyone experiences some type of skin concern at some point in their lives. Whether it's acne, wrinkles, dryness, or hyperpigmentation, these concerns can affect not only our physical appearance but also our mental and emotional well-being.

Each skin concern can have a significant impact on one's self-esteem and confidence, and it's crucial to understand the underlying causes and available solutions. Acne, for instance, affects up to fifty million Americans each year, and it can lead to scarring and post-inflammatory hyperpigmentation, thereby significantly impacting the social life of a person. Aging is another significant concern, as visible signs such as wrinkles, fine lines, and age spots can make us feel self-conscious and older than we are. Hyperpigmentation, dryness, and sensitivity can also cause discomfort and distress, and they are prevalent in people of all ages and skin types.

While there is no one-size-fits-all solution for these skin concerns, this chapter will cover some general principles and recommendations that can help you achieve healthier, clearer, and more radiant skin. We will discuss the common causes, symptoms, and prevention strategies for each concern, as well as the lifestyle changes that can make a difference. Whether you're struggling with a specific skin concern or looking to improve your overall skin health, this chapter will provide you with the knowledge and tools to make informed decisions about your skincare routine.

Acne

Acne is a common skin condition that affects people of all ages, but especially teenagers and young adults. Acne occurs due to clogging of the hair follicle openings with oil and dead skin cells. While acne is not a serious medical condition, it can be a source of embarrassment and anxiety for those who suffer from it.

Causes of Acne

There are several factors that can contribute to the development of acne. The most common cause is an overproduction of sebum, by the sebaceous glands in the skin. This can be due to hormonal changes, such as those that occur during puberty, menstruation, or pregnancy. Genetics can also play a role in the development of acne, as some people are simply more prone to the condition than others.

Build up of the dead skin cells can also contribute to the development of acne lesions. When these cells mix with sebum, they can form a plug in the hair follicle, which can lead to the development of a pimple. Bacteria (P. acnes) also play a role in the development of acne, as the bacteria that normally live on the skin can multiply in the clogged hair follicle and cause inflammation.

Treatment of Acne

There are several over-the-counter and prescription treatments that can be used to treat acne. The most commonly used over-the-counter treatments include benzoyl peroxide, salicylic acid, and alpha hydroxy acids. These treatments work by exfoliating the skin and unclogging the hair follicles, which can help to reduce the number of pimples and blackheads. They may also have antibacterial properties, which can help to reduce inflammation and prevent new breakouts from occurring.

Prescription treatments for acne include topical and oral medications. Topical antibiotics, such as clindamycin or erythromycin, can be used to reduce inflammation and kill bacteria on the skin. Topical retinoids, such as tretinoin or adapalene, can also be used to reduce inflammation and unclog hair follicles. Oral antibiotics, such as doxycycline or minocycline, can be used to treat pustular cases of acne.

In addition to medication, there are several procedures that can be used to treat acne. Chemical peels, which use a chemical solution to exfoliate the skin, can help to reduce the appearance of acne scars and prevent new breakouts. Laser therapy, which uses light to kill bacteria and reduce inflammation, can also be effective in treating acne.

It is best if you let your dermatologist choose the right treatment for you because many times self-medication can be harmful. With so much information at hand, many people get overconfident thinking that they can treat acne by themselves. Max was a teenager who struggled with acne. His classmates would make fun of his acne-prone face. Like many teenagers, he was self-conscious about his appearance and wanted to find a solution quickly. Max's parents were both busy with their professional life and couldn't pay much attention to his condition. To them, acne was not to be bothered about.

Many parents think that acne is just a part of adolescence and that with age they will settle down. They don't want to start treatment, especially in the initial phases of acne. They would want their child to first improve diet, exercise and try home remedies. While it is not bad to encourage your child for these things, you must realize that acne can have a significant impact on the mental or psychological well-being of your child. Studies have shown that early treatment for acne not only improves skin but increases the self-confidence of the person.

Max decided to take matters into his own hands. Max started reading about acne treatments online and stumbled upon a blog that recommended a particular over-the-counter cream. Without doing any further research, Max went to the drugstore and bought the cream. He started applying it to his face every night before bed, hoping to see some improvement.

After a few days, Max's skin started to become red and irritated. But, without realizing that concentration and duration of application of any cream are important, he didn't want to give up on the cream just yet, so he kept using it. Eventually, his skin became so inflamed and painful that he had to stay home from school. Max's parents became concerned and brought him to us. We discovered that Max was using a cream with a high concentration of benzoyl peroxide, which was too harsh for his sensitive skin.

Max's story is a cautionary tale about the dangers of self-medicating for skin conditions. While it's understandable to want to find a quick solution to a problem, it's important to consult with a healthcare professional before using any acne products on your skin. Doing so can save you a lot of pain, discomfort, and potential scarring.

Prevention of Acne

While there is no guaranteed way to prevent acne, there are several things that can be done to reduce the likelihood of developing it. The most important thing is to maintain a healthy skincare routine. This includes washing the face twice a day with a gentle cleanser, using oil-free and non-comedogenic makeup and skincare products, and avoiding touching the face with dirty hands. It is also important to avoid picking or squeezing pimples, as this can lead to scarring and further breakouts.

Diet can also play a role in the development of acne. While there is no clear consensus on which foods are most likely to cause acne, some studies have suggested that high-glycemic-index foods, such as sugary or starchy foods, may contribute to the development of acne. Eating a healthy, balanced diet that is rich in fruits, vegetables, and whole grains can help to reduce inflammation and keep the skin healthy. Finally, managing stress can also play a role in preventing acne. Stress can lead to increased oil production and acne breakouts. Stress reducing activities like meditation, yoga or exercise, can help to keep hormones in check and prevent acne from occurring.

If you have acne-prone skin, it is important to have a skincare routine that is specifically tailored to your skin type. Taking care of acne-prone skin requires a gentle and consistent skincare routine. By using the right products and avoiding harsh ingredients, you can help reduce breakouts and achieve clearer, healthier skin. Before we go to the next skin concern, let's see some of the habits that impact acne-prone skin:

Good Skin Habits

— Using a gentle cleanser: Wash your face with a gentle, non-comedogenic cleanser twice a day and avoid harsh cleansers which can agravate the acne lesions.

— Using products labeled as non-comedogenic: Look for products, such as moisturizers, sunscreens, and makeup, that are labeled as non-comedogenic, meaning they are formulated to not clog pores and cause acne.

- Exfoliating regularly: Use a gentle exfoliating product, such as a chemical exfoliant with alpha-hydroxy acids (AHAs) or beta-hydroxy acids (BHAs), to help remove dead skin cells and unclog pores.

- Keeping your hands off your face: Avoid touching your face, as this can transfer bacteria from your hands to your skin, leading to breakouts.

- Washing your pillowcase regularly: Dirty pillowcases can harbor bacteria and oil, so wash them regularly to help keep your skin clean.

- Using a spot treatment: Use a spot treatment containing benzoyl peroxide or salicylic acid to target individual pimples and help reduce inflammation.

- Moisturizing regularly: Even if your skin is oily, it still needs moisture. Look for a lightweight, oil-free moisturizer that won't clog pores.

- Protecting your skin from the sun: Use a broad-spectrum sunscreen with an SPF of 30 or higher to protect your skin from the sun's harmful rays. Sun damage can worsen acne and lead to scarring.

- Seeking professional help: If your acne is severe or not responding to over-the-counter treatments, consult a dermatologist for further treatment options.

Bad Skin Habits

- Picking at your skin: Resist the urge to pick or pop pimples, as this can lead to scarring and make acne worse.

- Using harsh skincare products: Avoid using harsh skincare products, such as toners containing alcohol, as these can irritate your skin and make acne worse.

— Overwashing or over-cleansing your face: Frequently washing your face can strip away the natural oils of skin and can lead to dry skin.

— Using oily products: Avoid using heavy, oily products, such as heavy creams or thick foundations, as they can clog pores and make acne worse.

— Skipping sunscreen: Sun damage can worsen acne and lead to scarring, so it's important to protect your skin from the sun's harmful rays with a broad-spectrum sunscreen.

— Using expired products: Expired skincare products can harbor bacteria and lead to breakouts, so always check the expiration date before using a product.

Hyperpigmentation

Hyperpigmentation is a common skin condition that affects many people. It occurs when there is an excess of melanin, the pigment that gives color to the skin, leading to the appearance of dark patches or spots. Hyperpigmentation can be caused by a variety of factors, such as sun exposure, hormonal changes, genetic factors, inflammatory disorders, skin allergies and skin injuries.

One of the most common types of hyperpigmentation we encounter in clinics is melasma. Melasma appears as gray-brown patches on the face, usually on the cheeks, forehead, nose, and upper lip. It is more common in women and is often triggered by hormonal changes, such as during pregnancy. Being most commonly present on the face, it affects the confidence of an individual. Age spots are caused by excessive sun exposure and usually appear on the hands, face and arms as flat, dark spots. Freckles are small, flat spots on the skin that are darker than the surrounding skin. They are usually genetic and appear most commonly on the face and arms. Post-inflammatory hyperpigmentation (PIH) is a type of hyperpigmentation that occurs after an injury or inflammation of the skin, such as acne, eczema, or a cut. PIH appears as flat, dark spots on the skin and can take months to fade.

Prevention

The first step in preventing hyperpigmentation is protecting the skin from the sun. Sun exposure is one of the primary causes of hyperpigmentation, especially in individuals with fair skin. The UV rays in sunlight stimulate the production of melanin in the skin, leading to dark spots and uneven skin tone. Therefore, it is essential to wear sunscreen daily to protect the skin from the sun's harmful rays.

Another way to prevent hyperpigmentation is to be gentle with your skin. Harsh scrubs and exfoliants can cause irritation and inflammation, which can lead to hyperpigmentation. Instead, opt for gentle cleansers and exfoliants that won't damage the skin's protective barrier. Also, avoid picking or squeezing pimples or other blemishes as this can cause inflammation and post-inflammatory hyperpigmentation.

A healthy diet is essential for maintaining healthy skin and preventing hyperpigmentation. Incorporating certain foods into your diet can provide the nutrients and antioxidants that your skin needs to function properly and prevent pigmentation issues. Here are some tips for creating a diet that can help prevent hyperpigmentation:

a. **Eat a Variety of Fruits and Vegetables:** Fruits and vegetables are rich in antioxidants, which can help protect the skin from damage caused by free radicals. Choose a variety of fruits and vegetables to ensure that you are getting a range of nutrients.

b. **Include Foods Rich in Vitamin C:** Vitamin C is essential for collagen production and helps to reduce the appearance of hyperpigmentation. Foods rich in vitamin C include citrus fruits, strawberries, kiwi, bell peppers, etc.

c. **Incorporate Foods with Vitamin E:** Vitamin E is a powerful antioxidant that helps to protect the skin from sun damage. Foods rich in vitamin E include nuts, seeds, avocados, and leafy greens.

d. **Eat Foods with Omega-3 Fatty Acids:** Omega-3 fatty acids can help reduce inflammation in the body, which can contribute to hyperpigmentation. Foods rich in omega-3s include fatty fish, nuts, and seeds.

e. **Avoid Processed and Sugary Foods:** Processed and sugary foods can contribute to inflammation in the body, which can exacerbate hyperpigmentation. Choose whole, nutrient-dense foods instead.

In addition to following a healthy diet, it is important to avoid smoking, drinking plenty of water also helps keep the skin hydrated, get enough sleep, and manage stress levels, as all of these factors can contribute to hyperpigmentation.

It is also essential to be mindful of the products you use on your skin. Certain skincare products can cause irritation and inflammation, which can lead to hyperpigmentation. David, a cabin crew, has to apply concealers and cosmetic products daily. David had always had a fair complexion, which he cherished. He believed that using various cosmetic products, vaguely, is not bad for the skin and so he kept on experimenting with different products. As time went by, David started noticing subtle changes in his skin. Dark patches began to appear on his cheeks, forehead, and even his neck. His skin started to become dry, itchy, and lustreless. At first, he dismissed it as a temporary effect of stress or fatigue, due to his hectic work schedule. But the hyperpigmentation and skin changes persisted and grew more prominent over time.

Little was he aware that if you don't maintain the natural balance of the skin, your skin starts to show subtle changes which might become prominent as time passes. Sometimes these skin changes are so slow to develop that people don't realize the cause.

Look for products that are gentle and formulated for your skin type. Avoid products that contain harsh chemicals, fragrances, or alcohol. It is also important to do a patch test before using a new product to ensure that it does not cause an adverse reaction.

Management of Hyperpigmentation

In addition to sunscreen, there are various topical treatments that can help fade hyperpigmentation. Hydroquinone, retinoids, and vitamin C, AHAs, BHAs are all effective in slowing down melanin production and promoting skin cell turnover. They are available in several concentrations and combinations. Several over-the-counter (OTC) brands and formulations claim to take away pigmentation but they are hardly successful in achieving what they claim. The lower concentration of active ingredients, improper quantity, and infrequent application, all can contribute to the ineffectiveness of these brands. Only a dermatologist can help you choose the proper formulation after accessing your pigmentation. Remember, pigmentation takes a long time to go away, patience is the key. There is no magic wand that can remove pigmentation overnight. Most people respond reasonably well if they follow the instructions provided by their dermatologist. Sometimes, even a good medical treatment might be ineffective and your dermatologist might recommend you several in-office procedures.

Chemical peels using alpha-hydroxy acids (AHAs) or beta-hydroxy acids (BHAs) can promote cell turnover and help fade hyperpigmentation. They are one of the common procedures being done in a dermatology setup. Choosing the right concentration and the right combination can reduce pigmentation in a faster and more effective way. Companies have started to enter this segment as well and are promoting home peels. But are they safe to be used at home?

One of our long-distance friends, Monai stumbled upon a DIY home peel brand. She was impressed by the way it was being promoted on the internet. She had heard about chemical peels in the past and how they can transform the skin. Without having any knowledge about the ingredients, she decided to give the brand a try for the pigmented spots on her face. As Monai waited for the facial peel to work its magic, she started to feel a tingling sensation on her skin. Initially, she brushed it off as a normal part of the process. But as time passed, the tingling turned into a burning sensation, and her face became red and inflamed.

Alarmed by the unexpected side effects, Monai quickly washed off the facial peel. However, the damage had already been done. Her skin was left sensitive, irritated, and covered in blotchy red patches. The patches turned black on next day as if the skin has been burned. She video-called us and showed her skin. We explained that the DIY facial peel she had used contained strong and potentially harsh ingredients that were too abrasive for her skin. The peel had caused a chemical burn and exacerbated her pigmentation issues.

Other modalities to treat hyperpigmentation includes laser therapy, medi facials, etc. However, all these treatments should only be performed by a licensed and experienced dermatologist.

Certain habits dictate the onset and outcomes in cases of hyperpigmentation:

Good Skin Habits

- Wearing sunscreen: Sunscreen is essential for preventing further hyperpigmentation and protecting your skin from UV rays.

- Using topical treatments: Topical treatments such as hydroquinone, retinoids, and vitamin C can help to reduce hyperpigmentation by slowing down melanin production and promoting skin cell turnover. Use these treatments as directed by your dermatologist.

- Exfoliating regularly: Regular exfoliation helps to remove dead skin cells and promote skin cell turnover, which can help to fade hyperpigmentation. Choose a gentle exfoliant and use it once or twice a week.

- Using a brightening serum: Brightening serums containing ingredients such as kojic acid or niacinamide can help to even out skin tone and reduce hyperpigmentation.

- Being patient: Hyperpigmentation can take time to fade, so be patient and stick to your skincare routine. Results may take several weeks or even months to become visible.

Bad Skin Habits

- Using harsh scrubs or exfoliants: Harsh scrubs or exfoliants can cause further irritation to the skin and exacerbate hyperpigmentation. Stick to gentle exfoliants instead.

- Picking at your skin: Picking at your skin can cause further damage and inflammation, leading to more hyperpigmentation. Avoid picking at pimples or other skin lesions.

- Using products containing irritants: Products containing ingredients such as alcohol, fragrances, or certain acids can cause irritation and inflammation, which can make hyperpigmentation worse. Check the labels of your skincare products and avoid anything that may cause irritation.

— Skipping sunscreen: Sun exposure can make hyperpigmentation worse, so it's essential to wear sunscreen every day, even when it's cloudy.

— Expecting immediate results: Hyperpigmentation can take time to fade, so don't expect immediate results from your skincare routine. Stick to your routine consistently and be patient.

Overall, managing hyperpigmentation requires a consistent and gentle skincare routine. By protecting your skin from the sun, using the right products, and avoiding harsh ingredients and habits, you can help to fade hyperpigmentation and achieve clearer, brighter skin.

Aging Skin

Aging skin is a natural process that occurs as a person grows older. It is characterized by a variety of changes in the skin's appearance and function, such as wrinkles, fine lines, thinning, dryness, and sagging. These changes occur due to a combination of factors including the loss of collagen and elastin, a decrease in the production of natural oils, and damage caused by environmental factors such as exposure to sunlight and pollution.

As we age, the skin's ability to repair itself also decreases, leading to slower wound healing and increased susceptibility to skin infections. The aging process can be accelerated by various lifestyle factors such as smoking, alcohol consumption, and poor diet.

It so often happens that confident person gets baffled when they start noticing the signs of aging on their skin. Sarah lives in a small town nestled near Delhi, and she had always been admired for her youthful appearance, with smooth and glowing skin that seemed to defy the passage of time.

As the years went by, Sarah reached her late forties, and she started to notice subtle changes in her skin. Fine lines began to form around her eyes and mouth, and her once firm complexion started to lose its elasticity. At first, Sarah shrugged off these changes, believing that she could easily reverse them with her usual skincare routine.

However, as time passed, Sarah's aging skin began to take a toll on her self-confidence. She found herself spending more and more time scrutinizing her reflection in the mirror, lamenting the loss of her youthful appearance. The once vibrant woman began to feel self-conscious and worried about what others might think of her.

Sarah's obsession with her aging skin soon became all-consuming. She started spending excessive amounts of money on various skincare products, hoping to find the magic solution that would turn back the clock. She eagerly tried every new fad and trend in the beauty industry, desperate to regain her youthful glow.

In her quest to reverse the signs of aging, Sarah also became isolated from her friends and family. She avoided social gatherings, fearing that others would notice and judge her changing appearance. Her once outgoing and confident personality became overshadowed by her fixation on her aging skin.

People don't embrace the natural process of aging and get into a panic situation very easily. Aging skin is just a natural part of life's journey, and it doesn't define anyone's worth as a person. Simultaneously, there is a lot you can do to delay or slow down the signs of skin aging.

One of the most important steps in preventing skin aging is protecting our skin from the sun. Sun exposure is a major factor in premature aging, as it damages the skin's collagen and elastin fibers, leading to sagging, wrinkles, and age spots. To protect your skin from the sun, it's important to wear a broad-spectrum sunscreen with an SPF of at least thirty every day, even on cloudy days. You should also wear protective clothing, such as long-sleeved shirts and hats, and avoid spending time in the sun during peak hours.

Targeted treatment options include the use of retinol, hyaluronic acid, peptides, and vitamin C serums. In-office treatment procedures are very popular these days as anti-aging modalities and include microdermabrasion, laser resurfacing, micro-needling radiofrequency, high-intensity focussed ultrasound, botulinum toxin, dermal fillers, PRP therapy, and mesotherapy.

Another important factor in preventing skin aging is maintaining a healthy lifestyle. Eating a antioxidants rich diet, such as fruits, vegetables, and whole grains, can help protect the skin from free radicals, which are unstable molecules that can damage skin cells and contribute to aging. A diet rich in nutrients and antioxidants can help to protect our skin from damage and keep it looking youthful and radiant.

Here are some of the key nutrients to include in your diet to prevent skin aging:

- **Vitamin C:** This powerful antioxidant helps to protect the skin from damage caused by UV radiation and pollution. It also plays a key role in collagen synthesis, which is important for maintaining the elasticity of the skin. Good sources of vitamin C include citrus fruits, berries, kiwi, and bell peppers.

- **Vitamin E:** Like vitamin C, vitamin E is an antioxidant that helps to protect the skin from damage caused by free radicals. It also helps to improve the skin's moisture barrier, which can help to prevent dryness and wrinkles. Good sources of vitamin E include nuts, seeds, and leafy green vegetables.

- **Omega-3 Fatty Acids:** These essential fatty acids are important for maintaining the health of the skin's cell membranes, which can help to prevent damage and inflammation. Good sources of omega-3s include fatty fish such as salmon and sardines, as well as flaxseeds, chia seeds, and walnuts.

- **Carotenoids:** These pigments give colors to fruits and vegetables and also have antioxidant properties that can help to protect the skin from damage. Good sources of carotenoids include carrots, sweet potatoes, tomatoes, and spinach.

- **Water:** Staying hydrated is crucial for maintaining the health and appearance of the skin

Here are some of the habits that led to good skin aging vs bad skin aging:

Good Skin Habits

- Using a gentle cleanser to avoid stripping the skin of its natural oils.

- Using a moisturizer that contains antioxidants and other beneficial ingredients to help protect the skin from damage.

- Applying sunscreen daily to protect the skin from the harmful effects of UV radiation.

- Using products that contain retinoids or other anti-aging ingredients, as these can help improve the appearance of fine lines and wrinkles.

- Staying hydrated by drinking plenty of water and eating a diet rich in fruits and vegetables.

- Getting enough sleep allows the skin time to repair and regenerate.

- Exercising regularly to improve circulation and promote healthy skin.

Bad Skin Habits

- Using harsh soaps or scrubs, which can damage the skin.

- Using hot water when washing your face or taking a shower, as this can dry out the skin.

- Smoking, as can accelerate the aging process and cause damage to the skin.

- Excessive alcohol consumption, as it can dehydrate the skin and contribute to the development of wrinkles.

- Forgetting to remove makeup before going to bed, as leaving it on can clog pores and lead to breakouts.

- Using tanning beds, as they can damage the skin and increase the risk of skin cancer.

- Stress, as it can contribute to the development of wrinkles and other signs of aging.

SECTION SIX

Lifestyle and Skincare

SECTION SIX

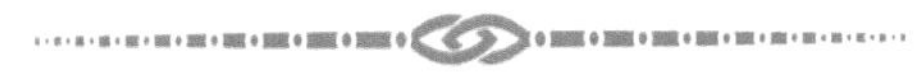

Lifestyle and Skincare

Exploring the Harmonious Balance

Skincare is not just about applying products to your face; it's a reflection of your lifestyle habits. What you eat, how much you sleep, and how you manage your stress all affect your skin's health and appearance. Sometimes, despite using the best skincare products, the skin changes that you expect are not achieved. Many a time, when we take the history of such people, there is always a lifestyle-related factor (or more than one) that is halting the skincare goals.

Milani was an air-hostess and had always struggled with her skin. Despite using good skincare products and consulting some of the best dermatologists, she was frustrated and longing for clear and radiant skin. Now and then, she would have some skin issues. After attending one of our seminars for a cabin-crew training institute, she understood the role of lifestyle changes in skin health.

Milani began by examining her diet. She realized that she often indulged in processed foods, sugary snacks, and unhealthy drinks. Determined to make a change, she started incorporating more fruits, vegetables, and whole grains into her meals. She also made sure to drink plenty of water to keep her skin hydrated from within.

Along with improving her diet, Milani recognized the importance of regular exercise. She discovered that physical activity not only helped her maintain a healthy weight but also improved her circulation and brought a natural glow to her skin. She incorporated different forms of exercise into her routine, from jogging and yoga to dance classes, finding joy and fulfillment in being active.

Stress was another factor that Milani identified as a possible contributor to her skin woes. She realized that her hectic lifestyle and constant worries were taking a toll on her complexion. To combat this, she incorporated stress management techniques into her daily life. Milani began practicing mindfulness and meditation, carving out time each day to relax and unwind. This newfound focus on mental well-being not only helped alleviate her stress but also reflected positively on her skin.

As Milani continued to make positive lifestyle changes, she noticed a significant improvement in her skin. Her complexion became clearer, more radiant, and had a healthy glow. Friends and family started complimenting her on her vibrant appearance, and Milani couldn't help but feel a sense of pride and accomplishment.

Milani's journey not only transformed her skin but also transformed her outlook on life. She realized that true beauty came from taking care of oneself, both inside and out. By making positive lifestyle changes, she had not only achieved great skin but had also discovered a newfound confidence and self-love.

Healthy Diet

Your skin is the largest organ, and what you eat can have a significant impact on your health. A diet rich in fruits, vegetables, lean protein, and healthy fats can provide your skin with the nutrients it needs to stay healthy. Vitamin C, for example, can help boost collagen production, while omega-3 fatty acids can help keep your skin hydrated and supple.

On the other hand, a diet high in sugar and processed foods can lead to inflammation, which can contribute to acne and other skin conditions. Some foods especially, dairy products like milk, cheese, and yogurt can trigger acne in some people. They may contain hormones and growth factors that can increase oil production and inflammation in the skin.

To improve your skin's health, focus on eating a healthy, balanced diet that includes plenty of whole foods. Though it is impossible to discuss the entire list of foods, below we have listed some examples of foods that are good and bad for skin health.

Good Food for Skin

- **Fatty Fish:** Fatty fish is rich in omega-3 fatty acids, which help nourish the skin and keep it supple. Omega-3s also have anti-inflammatory properties that can alleviate skin conditions like acne and eczema.

- **Avocados:** Avocados are packed with healthy fats, vitamin E, and antioxidants. These nutrients help moisturize and protect the skin from oxidative damage. They also support collagen production, which contributes to skin elasticity.

- **Berries:** Blueberries, strawberries, and other berries are excellent sources of antioxidants. Antioxidants combat free radicals and help prevent premature aging. Berries are also rich in vitamin C, which aids in collagen synthesis and promotes a youthful complexion.

- **Nuts and Seeds:** Almonds, walnuts, flaxseeds, and chia seeds are all beneficial for the skin. They contain omega-3 fatty acids, vitamin E, and zinc, which help maintain skin integrity and reduce inflammation.

- **Sweet Potatoes:** Sweet potatoes are high in beta-carotene, which converts to vitamin A in the body. Vitamin A is essential for healthy skin, as it promotes cell turnover and helps protect against sun damage.

- **Leafy Greens:** Spinach, kale, and other leafy greens are packed with vitamins, minerals, and antioxidants. They provide nutrients like vitamin C, vitamin E, and beta-carotene, which are all crucial for skin health and repair.

- **Tomatoes:** Tomatoes are an excellent source of lycopene, an antioxidant that helps protect the skin from sun damage and enhances its natural defense against UV rays. They also contain vitamin C, which aids collagen production.

- **Green Tea:** Green tea is known for its high content of antioxidants called catechins. These compounds help protect the skin from sun damage and reduce inflammation. Drinking green tea regularly can contribute to a healthier complexion.

- **Citrus Fruits:** Oranges, lemons, grapefruits, and other citrus fruits are rich in vitamin C, which is essential for collagen synthesis. Vitamin C also acts as an antioxidant, protecting the skin from oxidative stress and supporting a brighter complexion.

- **Dark Chocolate:** Good news for chocolate lovers! Dark chocolate with a high cocoa content contains antioxidants called flavonoids, which can improve skin hydration, and texture, and protect against sun damage. Remember to choose dark chocolate with a minimum of seventy percent cocoa for optimal benefits.

- **Bell Peppers:** Bell peppers, particularly the red and yellow varieties, are abundant in vitamin C and antioxidants. These nutrients help protect the skin from environmental damage and contribute to a more youthful appearance.

- **Turmeric:** Turmeric is known for its anti-inflammatory properties. Curcumin, the active compound in turmeric, has been shown to reduce skin inflammation and promote healing. Adding turmeric to your meals or enjoying a cup of turmeric tea can be beneficial for your skin.

- **Greek Yogurt:** Greek yogurt is an excellent source of protein and probiotics. Protein is necessary for collagen synthesis, while probiotics support a healthy gut microbiome, which can impact skin health. Opt for plain, unsweetened Greek yogurt for the best results.

- **Olive Oil:** Olive oil is rich in healthy fats and antioxidants, including vitamin E. These components help moisturize and protect the skin from oxidative stress, maintaining its elasticity and promoting a more youthful appearance. Use olive oil as a dressing or for cooking instead of less healthy oils.

- **Watermelon:** Watermelon is not only a refreshing summer fruit but also hydrating for the skin. It contains vitamins A and C, which are vital for skin health and hydration.

- **Pumpkin Seeds:** Pumpkin seeds are rich in zinc, which plays a crucial role in regulating oil production and promoting skin healing. They also contain antioxidants and essential fatty acids that support overall skin health.

- **Broccoli:** Broccoli is packed with vitamins A, C, and E, as well as antioxidants. These nutrients help protect the skin from damage, promote collagen production, and contribute to a clear and radiant complexion.

- **Kiwi:** Kiwi is a fruit that's bursting with vitamin C, which is important for collagen synthesis and maintaining skin elasticity. It also contains other essential nutrients like vitamin E and antioxidants that support skin health.

- **Oats:** Oats are a great source of fiber and contain compounds that have anti-inflammatory properties. They can help soothe irritated skin and provide relief for conditions like eczema. Oats also contain vitamins and minerals that support overall skin health.

- **Red Grapes:** Red grapes are rich in resveratrol, a powerful antioxidant that helps protect the skin from damage and fights signs of aging. They also contain natural fruit acids that can improve skin tone and texture.

- **Eggs:** Eggs are a good source of protein, which is essential for collagen production and promoting skin elasticity. They also contain biotin, a B-vitamin that contributes to healthy skin, hair, and nails.

- **Carrots:** Carrots have beta-carotene, which converts to vitamin A in the body. Vitamin A is necessary for healthy skin, as it promotes cell turnover and helps protect against dryness and wrinkles.

- **Garlic:** Garlic has antibacterial and anti-inflammatory properties that can benefit the skin, particularly for acne-prone individuals. It also contains sulfur, which promotes collagen production and supports a healthy complexion.

- **Brazil Nuts:** Brazil nuts contains selenium, an antioxidant mineral that helps protect the skin from sun damage and maintain its elasticity. They also provide healthy fats and vitamin E for nourished skin.

- **Water:** Staying hydrated is essential for healthy skin. Drinking plenty of water helps keep the skin moisturized, flushes out toxins, and supports healthy digestion and elimination.

Bad Foods for Skin

- **Processed Foods:** Highly processed foods, such as fast food, sugary snacks, and packaged snacks, often contain high amounts of refined carbohydrates, unhealthy fats, and additives. These ingredients may contribute to inflammation in the body, which can manifest as skin issues like acne and breakouts.

- **Artificial Trans Fats:** Artificial trans fats, commonly found in processed and fried foods, have been associated with increased inflammation and a higher risk of acne. These unhealthy fats can also contribute to a dull complexion and accelerate skin aging.

- **Sugar:** Excessive sugar and high-glycemic foods can lead to increased inflammation and insulin spikes. This can trigger the production of sebum and contribute to the development of acne. Additionally, a high-sugar diet may accelerate the breakdown of collagen, leading to premature skin aging.

- **Refined Grains:** Refined grains, such as white bread, white rice, and pasta made from refined flour, have a high glycemic index. These foods can cause a rapid spike in blood sugar levels, potentially triggering inflammation and exacerbating skin conditions like acne.

- **Dairy Products:** Though dairy products are well tolerated by many people and are considered very good dietary supplements, high-fat dairy products have been associated with an increased risk of acne in some individuals. It is thought that the hormones present in dairy, as well as its potential inflammatory properties, may contribute to skin issues for certain people.

- **Fried and Greasy Foods:** Foods that are deep-fried or cooked in unhealthy oils can be detrimental to skin health. These foods are often high in unhealthy fats, which can lead to increased oil production and clogged pores. This can result in acne breakouts and dull-looking skin.

- **Saturated Fats:** Consuming excessive amounts of saturated fats, which are found in dairy products, fatty cuts of meat, and some processed foods, can contribute to inflammation in the body. This inflammation may manifest as skin issues like acne and eczema.

- **Artificial Sweeteners:** Artificial sweeteners, often found in diet sodas, sugar-free snacks, and some low-calorie desserts, can potentially disrupt the balance of gut bacteria and contribute to inflammation. This gut-skin connection may lead to skin issues for some individuals.

- **Processed Meats:** Processed meats often contain additives, preservatives, and high levels of sodium. These ingredients can contribute to inflammation and potentially worsen skin conditions.

- **Excessive Alcohol:** Consuming excessive amounts of alcohol can dehydrate the body and lead to dull and dry skin. Alcohol also widens blood vessels, potentially causing redness and inflammation. Over time, excessive alcohol consumption can contribute to premature aging and worsen certain skin conditions.

- **Caffeine and Excessive Coffee:** While moderate caffeine consumption is generally fine for most people, excessive intake can dehydrate the body and potentially worsen skin dryness.

Additionally, some individuals may find that caffeine triggers or exacerbates skin conditions like acne.

- **Gluten and Potential Sensitivities:** For individuals with gluten sensitivities or celiac disease, consuming gluten-containing foods can trigger inflammation and various skin conditions like eczema or dermatitis herpetiformis.

- **High-Sodium Foods:** Foods rich in sodium, such as processed meats, canned soups, and salty snacks, can contribute to water retention and puffiness. This can make the skin appear swollen and potentially worsen the appearance of under-eye bags.

- **High-Fructose Corn Syrup:** High-fructose corn syrup, a common sweetener in some foods and beverages, has been linked to increased inflammation and insulin resistance. These effects can potentially worsen skin conditions like acne and contribute to premature skin aging.

- **Spicy Foods:** Spicy foods can cause blood vessels in the skin to dilate, leading to facial redness and flushing. In some individuals, spicy foods can trigger or worsen conditions like rosacea.

Sleep

Getting enough sleep (on average six to eight hours per day) is essential for good health, and it's also critical for healthy skin. While you sleep, your skin repairs itself, and new skin cells are produced. Lack of sleep can lead to dark circles, puffy eyes, and a dull complexion. Additionally, chronic sleep deprivation can increase your stress levels, which can contribute to skin problems such as acne and eczema. Similarly, excessive sleep can also have a negative impact on skin health. Oversleeping can contribute to fluid retention in the body, including the face. This can lead to morning puffiness and a bloated appearance of the skin, particularly around the eyes and cheeks. Lack of movement and exposure to air-conditioners during prolonged periods of sleep can also contribute to skin dehydration. Excessive sleep can disrupt the skin's natural balance. It may lead to increased oil production, clogged pores, and the potential for breakouts, particularly if you're not cleansing your face properly before going to bed.

Some potential impacts of insufficient sleep or chronic sleep deprivation include:

- **Dark Circles and Under-Eye Bags:** Lack of sleep can cause blood vessels under the eyes to dilate, resulting in the appearance of dark circles and under-eye bags. Reduced sleep can also lead to fluid retention, making the under-eye area appear puffy and swollen.

- **Dull Complexion:** Sleep deprivation can affect the skin's natural radiance and lead to a dull complexion. Inadequate sleep disrupts the skin's ability to repair and regenerate, resulting in a lackluster appearance and decreased skin vitality.

- **Increased Signs of Aging:** Chronic sleep deprivation can accelerate the aging process and contribute to the formation of fine lines, wrinkles, and uneven skin texture. During sleep, the body releases growth hormone, which aids in the repair and regeneration of skin cells. Insufficient sleep can disrupt this process, leading to premature aging.

- **Skin Sensitivity and Irritation:** Lack of sleep can compromise the skin's barrier function, making it more susceptible to external irritants. This can result in increased skin sensitivity, redness, and irritation, making existing skin conditions like acne, eczema, or psoriasis worse.

- **Impaired Skin Healing:** Sleep is a critical time for the body to repair and regenerate tissues, including the skin. Inadequate sleep can impair the skin's ability to heal from wounds, breakouts, or other skin issues, prolonging their recovery time.

- **Increased Inflammation:** Lack of sleep triggers a stress response in the body, leading to increased production of stress hormones like cortisol. Elevated cortisol levels can contribute to inflammation in the body, including the skin. This inflammation can exacerbate existing skin conditions or trigger flare-ups.

- **Imbalanced Skin Functions:** Sleep deprivation can disrupt the delicate balance of skin functions, such as oil production and hydration. This imbalance can lead to increased sebum production, clogged pores, and the development of acne.

How to Improve Sleep Quality?

Quality sleep is vital for overall health and well-being. However, many individuals struggle with achieving restful and rejuvenating sleep. Though discussing the sleep cycle and its quality is out of the scope of this book, there are various effective strategies for improving sleep quality, including establishing a consistent sleep routine, creating a sleep-friendly environment, adopting relaxation techniques, and practicing healthy lifestyle habits.

Establish a Consistent Sleep Routine

Creating a regular sleep schedule helps regulate the body's internal clock, promoting better sleep quality. Aim to go to bed and wake up at the same time every day, even on weekends. This consistency helps synchronize the sleep-wake cycle, making it easier to fall asleep and wake up naturally.

Create a Sleep-Friendly Environment

Optimize your sleep environment to promote relaxation and minimize disturbances. Ensure your bedroom is dark, quiet, and cool. Consider using blackout curtains, earplugs, or white noise machines to block out external stimuli. Choose a comfortable mattress, pillows, and bedding that support your preferred sleeping position.

Adopt Relaxation Techniques

Engage in relaxation techniques before bedtime to signal to your body that it's time to unwind and prepare for sleep. These techniques can include deep breathing exercises, progressive muscle relaxation, meditation, or gentle stretching. Avoid stimulating activities, such as intense exercise or using electronic devices, close to bedtime.

Practice Good Sleep Hygiene

Developing healthy sleep habits can significantly improve sleep quality. Some practices to consider include avoiding caffeine and heavy meals in the evening, limiting alcohol consumption, and avoiding nicotine. Establish a wind-down routine before bed that includes relaxing activities, such as reading a book, taking a warm bath, or practicing a calming hobby.

Create a Technology-Free Zone

The blue light emitted by electronic devices can interfere with sleep quality. Establish a technology-free zone in your bedroom by removing TVs, smartphones, tablets, and other screens. Avoid using electronic devices for at least an hour before bedtime to allow your brain to transition into a state of relaxation.

Limit Daytime Napping

While short power naps can be refreshing, excessive daytime napping can disrupt night-time sleep. If you struggle with sleep quality, limit daytime naps to twenty to thirty minutes and avoid napping too close to bedtime. This helps maintain a proper sleep-wake balance.

Engage in Regular Physical Activity

Regular exercise promotes better sleep quality by reducing stress, increasing sleep efficiency, and improving overall well-being. Engage in moderate-intensity physical activity, such as brisk walking or yoga, for at least thirty minutes most days of the week. However, avoid exercising too close to bedtime, as it can energize the body and make it harder to fall asleep.

Manage Stress and Worry

Persistent stress and worry can interfere with sleep. Establish effective stress management techniques, such as practicing mindfulness, journaling, or seeking support from a therapist. Create a relaxing bedtime routine that helps clear your mind and prepares you for restful sleep.

Stress

Stress is an unavoidable part of life, and its impact extends beyond mental and emotional well-being. There is a complex relationship between the mind and the skin. There are many physiological responses triggered by stress and they can manifest in various skin conditions. When you're stressed, your body produces cortisol, a hormone that can cause inflammation, which can exacerbate skin conditions like acne and eczema. Additionally, stress can cause you to neglect your skincare routine, leading to clogged pores and breakouts.

Acne Breakouts

Stress can stimulate the production of stress hormones like cortisol, which can lead to an increase in sebum (oil) production. Excessive sebum, along with dead skin cells, can clog pores and contribute to the development of acne breakouts. Stress-induced acne is often characterized by inflammatory and persistent lesions.

Skin Sensitivity and Irritation

Stress weakens the skin's natural barrier function, making it more susceptible to external irritants. This can lead to heightened skin sensitivity, redness, itching, and even allergic reactions. Individuals may find that their skin reacts more strongly to skincare products, environmental pollutants, or other triggers during periods of elevated stress.

Premature Aging

Chronic stress accelerates the aging process and can contribute to the development of premature signs of aging. Increased production of cortisol and other stress hormones can break down collagen and elastin fibers in the skin, leading to a loss of elasticity, fine lines, wrinkles, and a dull complexion. Additionally, stress-induced oxidative damage can further exacerbate the aging process.

Impaired Skin Healing

Stress disrupts the normal healing process of the skin, making it more difficult for wounds, injuries, or skin conditions to heal properly. The compromised immune function associated with stress can prolong the recovery time of skin ailments, such as cuts, abrasions, or inflammatory conditions like eczema or psoriasis.

Worsening of Existing Skin Conditions

Stress can exacerbate existing skin conditions. Conditions like eczema, psoriasis, rosacea, or dermatitis may flare up or become more difficult to manage during times of stress. Stress weakens the immune system, triggers inflammation, and disrupts the skin's natural balance, aggravating these chronic skin conditions.

Impaired Barrier Function

Stress can compromise the skin's protective barrier function, making it more prone to dehydration and moisture loss. This can result in dryness, flakiness, and an overall compromised skin barrier. A weakened skin barrier allows irritants and allergens to penetrate more easily, leading to further skin problems.

Overall, stress has a profound impact on skin health. Understanding the complex relationship between stress and skin is essential for adopting effective stress management techniques and maintaining optimal skin health. By prioritizing stress reduction strategies, such as practicing relaxation techniques, engaging in regular exercise, seeking social support, and adopting a balanced lifestyle, individuals can mitigate the negative effects of stress on their skin and promote overall well-being.

Remember, skincare is not just about the products you use; it's about the lifestyle choices you make every day. Your lifestyle habits can have a significant impact on the health and appearance of your skin. By eating a healthy diet, getting enough sleep, managing stress, and protecting your skin from the sun, you can improve your skin's health and reduce your risk of developing skin problems like acne and premature aging.

Skincare for Different Ages

SECTION SEVEN

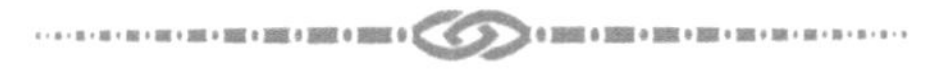

Skincare for Different Ages

Healthy Skin is Timeless

Skincare is an essential part of our daily routine, and it becomes increasingly important as we age. As we get older, our skin undergoes changes that require us to adjust our skincare regimen. Let us try to see what physiological changes happen in our skin and how our skincare regimens change.

In the early phases of adolescence and young adulthood, hormonal changes cause a whirlwind of emotions and transformations. The skin becomes a battleground for excess sebum production, leading to oily skin and pesky acne breakouts. Gentle cleansing rituals become the knights in shining armor, battling against the onslaught of excess oil. Exfoliation, like a loyal companion, steps forward to unclog pores and restore balance. And the quest for non-comedogenic products becomes a sacred mission to prevent further breakouts and protect delicate young skin.

As the story progresses into the next phases of early to mid-adulthood, the skin faces a new adversary—time. Collagen and elastin, the pillars of youth, begin their gradual descent, leaving behind fine lines and wrinkles as evidence of their fading power.

Skincare regimens transform into a battlefield of anti-aging weapons. Retinoids, the potent warriors, fight to stimulate collagen production and reduce the appearance of fine lines. Antioxidants, like magical spells, cast protection against free radicals and environmental damage. And peptides, the secret agents, stealthily work to enhance elasticity and firmness. The hero of sunscreen emerges, shielding the skin from the harmful rays of the sun, a relentless enemy of youthful skin.

The tale moves into the phases of mature adulthood, where the battle against time intensifies. Collagen and elastin continue their retreat, leaving the skin with deeper wrinkles and sagging. Dryness and sensitivity enter the scene, as the skin's ability to retain moisture dwindles. Skincare regimens shift their focus to deep hydration and intense moisturization in addition to retinoids. Hyaluronic acid, the magical elixir, quenches the skin's thirst and plumps up its appearance. Ceramides, the fortifiers, restore the skin's natural moisture barrier, ensuring it remains strong and resilient. And rich, nourishing creams become the knights in shining armor, providing the necessary armor against dryness and promoting a supple complexion.

The final phases unfold in the realm of seniorhood, where a whole new set of challenges emerges. Hormonal fluctuations (for females) wreak havoc on the skin, leaving it parched, thin, and lacking density. Skincare regimens become an oasis of hydration, with emollients, humectants, and occlusives working together to replenish the skin's moisture stores. Phytoestrogens, like ancient remedies, soothe the skin and promote collagen production, breathing life into the fading complexion. The use of retinoids and hyaluronic acid (and other moisturizers) continues.

Through the understanding of the skin's ever-evolving physiology, individuals are able to adapt their skincare rituals to the changing needs of each chapter in their lives.

Teenagers (thirteen to nineteen years)

Teenagers are at a crucial stage in their lives when it comes to skincare. This is the time when hormones are raging, and acne is a common problem. It is important to develop healthy habits at this age that will benefit the skin in the long run.

- **Cleanse:** Start with a gentle cleanser that removes excess oil and dirt from the skin. Avoid using harsh scrubs that can damage the skin and cause more breakouts.

- **Moisturize:** Use a light moisturizer that is oil-free and non-comedogenic. This will help keep the skin hydrated without clogging pores.

- **Sunscreen:** Apply a broad-spectrum sunscreen. This will help protect the skin from harmful UV rays.

- **Avoid Touching the Face:** Keep hands away from the face as much as possible to avoid spreading bacteria that can cause breakouts.

- **Seek help for breakouts**: Avoid self-medication and visit a dermatologist for acne and other skin issues.

Twenties to Thirties

In your twenties and thirties, your skin is still youthful and vibrant, but it is also the time when fine lines and wrinkles start to appear. It is important to establish a skincare routine that helps prevent premature aging.

- **Cleanse:** Use a gentle cleanser to remove dirt and makeup from the skin.

- **Exfoliate:** Use a gentle exfoliator once or twice a week to remove dead skin cells and promote cell turnover.

- **Moisturize:** Use a moisturizer that is suitable for your skin type to keep the skin hydrated and plump.

- **Sunscreen:** Apply a broad-spectrum sunscreen with an SPF of at least 30 every day to protect the skin from UV damage.

- **Eye Cream:** Use an eye cream that contains antioxidants and peptides to help reduce the appearance of fine lines and wrinkles.

- **Antioxidants:** Use products that contain antioxidants like vitamin C and E to help protect the skin from free radical damage.

- **Retinoids:** Use products that contain retinoids to help reduce the appearance of fine lines and wrinkles.

Forties to Fifties

In your forties and fifties, the skin starts to lose elasticity, and wrinkles become more prominent. It is important to use products that help improve skin firmness and texture.

- **Cleanse:** Use a gentle cleanser that does not strip the skin of its natural oils.

- **Exfoliate:** Use a gentle exfoliator once or twice a week to promote cell turnover and improve skin texture.

- **Moisturize:** Use a moisturizer that contains hyaluronic acid to help hydrate the skin and improve skin firmness.

- **Sunscreen:** Apply a broad-spectrum sunscreen with an SPF of at least 30 every day to protect the skin from further damage.

- **Retinoids:** Use products that contain retinoids to help reduce the appearance of fine lines and wrinkles.

- **Peptides:** Use products that contain peptides to help improve skin firmness and elasticity.

- **Vitamin C:** Use products that contain vitamin C to help brighten the skin and improve skin texture.

- **Eye Cream:** Use an eye cream that contains retinol and antioxidants to help reduce the appearance of fine lines and wrinkles.

Beyond Fifties

As we age, our skin becomes thinner and more fragile, which can lead to wrinkles, age spots, and dryness. In order to maintain healthy skin in your fifties and beyond, it's important to use a skincare regimen that focuses on improving skin density and hydration. Here are some tips and products to consider:

- **Cleanse:** Use a gentle cleanser that does not strip the skin of its natural oils. Look for products that are formulated for mature skin and contain moisturizing ingredients like hyaluronic acid or glycerine.

- **Exfoliate:** Use a gentle exfoliator once or twice a week to promote cell turnover and improve skin texture. Look for products that contain alpha hydroxy acids (AHAs) or beta hydroxy acids (BHAs), which can help slough off dead skin cells and stimulate collagen production.

- **Moisturize:** Use a moisturizer that contains nourishing ingredients like ceramides, peptides, and antioxidants to help hydrate and strengthen the skin. Look for products that are specifically formulated for mature skin, as they tend to be more emollient and have a richer texture.

- **Sunscreen:** Apply a broad-spectrum sunscreen with an SPF of at least 30 every day to protect the skin from further damage.

Look for products that contain zinc oxide or titanium dioxide, which provide physical protection against the sun's harmful UV rays.

- **Retinoids:** Use products that contain retinoids to help reduce the appearance of fine lines and wrinkles. Retinoids are a form of vitamin A that can help stimulate collagen production and improve skin texture. However, they can also be irritating to the skin, so it's important to start with a low concentration and gradually increase over time.

- **Peptides:** Use products that contain peptides to help improve skin firmness and elasticity. Peptides are short chains of amino acids that can help stimulate collagen production and improve skin texture.

- **Vitamin C:** Use products that contain vitamin C to help brighten the skin and improve skin texture. Vitamin C is a powerful antioxidant that can help protect the skin from free radical damage and promote collagen production.

- **Eye Cream:** Use an eye cream that contains retinol and antioxidants to help reduce the appearance of fine lines and wrinkles. Look for products that also contain caffeine, which can help reduce puffiness and dark circles around the eyes.

Skincare for Different Skin Types

SECTION EIGHT

Skincare for Different Skin Types

Unique Skin, Unique Care

In terms of skin physiology, each skin type tells a unique tale. From oily to dry, sensitive to combination, the intricacies of skin physiology vary, shaping the needs and challenges faced by individuals. Let's explore the fascinating world of skin types and their distinct characteristics.

Oily skin, like a well-scripted drama, is known for its overactive sebaceous glands. These glands produce an excess of sebum, leading to a shiny complexion and a predisposition to acne breakouts. The skin's natural lipid barrier may be disrupted, making it more susceptible to environmental aggressors. Skincare for oily skin focuses on gentle cleansing to remove excess oil, oil-free or lightweight moisturizers to maintain hydration without clogging pores, and the use of non-comedogenic products to prevent further breakouts.

Dry skin, akin to a poetic sonnet, lacks sufficient moisture and may experience tightness, flakiness, and dullness. It may appear rough and feel rough to the touch. The skin's lipid barrier is compromised, leading to increased transepidermal water loss (TEWL). Skincare for dry skin revolves around deep hydration and replenishment. It involves the use of creamy cleansers, rich moisturizers with emollients and humectants to lock in moisture, and gentle exfoliation to remove dead skin cells.

Combination skin, a tale of duality, exhibits characteristics of both oily and dry skin. The T-zone, consisting of the forehead, nose, and chin, tends to be oilier, while the cheeks may lean towards dryness. This skin type requires a delicate balancing act. Skincare for combination skin involves a targeted approach. It may include using a gentle cleanser to control excess oil in the T-zone, lightweight moisturizers for dry areas, and products that cater to specific concerns in each zone.

Sensitive skin, like a fragile porcelain figurine, is prone to react adversely to various environmental and chemical factors. It may display redness, irritation, and a heightened response to skincare products or environmental triggers. The skin's barrier function is compromised, allowing irritants to penetrate more easily. Skincare for sensitive skin centers around soothing and calming ingredients. It involves using mild, fragrance-free cleansers, hypoallergenic and non-irritating products, and avoiding harsh ingredients like fragrances, alcohol, and certain preservatives.

Understanding the unique characteristics of different skin types allows for tailored skincare regimens. It enables individuals to address their specific concerns while maintaining optimal skin health. Whether battling excess oil, combating dryness, seeking balance, or soothing sensitivity, the intricate dance of skin physiology guides individuals on their skincare journey. By embracing the individuality of their skin type, individuals can script their own narrative of beauty and well-being, nurturing their skin with care and precision.

Normal Skin

If you have normal skin, congratulations! Your skin is well-balanced and generally not prone to sensitivity, dryness, or oiliness. However, it's still important to take care of your skin to keep it healthy and glowing. Here is a skincare regimen and some recommended products for normal skin:

- **Cleanser:** Use a gentle cleanser twice a day to remove dirt, oil, and makeup. Look for a cleanser that is pH-balanced and free of harsh chemicals or fragrances.

- **Toner:** Use a toner to balance the pH of your skin and help prepare it for other products. Look for a toner that is alcohol-free and contains soothing ingredients like aloe vera or chamomile.

- **Moisturizer:** Use a lightweight moisturizer to keep your skin hydrated and protected. Look for a moisturizer that is non-comedogenic and free of heavy oils or fragrances.

- **Sunscreen:** Use a broad-spectrum sunscreen with an SPF of at least 30 every day to protect your skin from the sun's harmful rays. Look for a sunscreen that is non-greasy and won't leave a white cast on your skin.

- **Exfoliator:** Exfoliating once or twice a week can help remove dead skin cells and promote cell turnover, revealing brighter, smoother skin. Look for a gentle exfoliator that won't irritate your skin or cause micro-tears.

- **Face Mask:** Using a face mask once a week can help boost your skin's hydration and radiance. Look for a face mask that contains nourishing ingredients like hyaluronic acid, antioxidants, or vitamin C.

Good Skin Habits

- Cleansing your skin twice daily using a gentle cleanser to remove dirt, oil, and makeup.

- Using a toner after cleansing to restore your skin's pH balance and prepare it for moisturization.

- Moisturizing daily to maintain your skin's hydration and prevent dryness or flakiness.

- Using a sunscreen with at least SPF 30 daily to protect your skin from harmful UV rays.

- Exfoliating your skin once or twice a week to remove dead skin cells and promote cell turnover.

- Drinking plenty of water and eat a healthy, balanced diet to nourish your skin from within.

Bad Skin Habits

- Using harsh or abrasive scrubs, peels, or exfoliants (they can damage your skin and cause irritation)

- Using too many products at once (this can overwhelm your skin and disrupt its natural balance)

- Using hot water to cleanse your skin (it can strip away your skin's natural oils and cause dryness)

- Forgetting to remove your makeup before going to bed (it can clog your pores and cause breakouts)

- Touching your face too often (this can transfer bacteria and oils from your hands onto your skin)

- Forgetting to get enough sleep (lack of sleep can affect your skin's appearance and cause dark circles)

Oily Skin

If you have oily skin, you may be more prone to breakouts, clogged pores, and shiny skin. It's essential to maintain a proper skincare routine to balance the oil production in your skin and prevent these issues. Here's a skincare regime you can try for oily skin:

- **Cleanse:** Start by washing your face twice a day with a gentle cleanser formulated for oily skin. Look for products that contain salicylic acid, benzoyl peroxide, or glycolic acid, which can help to unclog pores and control excess oil production.

- **Tone:** After cleansing, use a toner that's specifically formulated for oily skin to help remove any remaining dirt and oil from your pores. Witch hazel, tea tree oil, and aloe vera are some ingredients that can be helpful in reducing oil and calming inflammation.

- **Moisturize:** Moisturizing is still important even for oily skin types. Choose a lightweight, oil-free moisturizer that won't clog your pores. Look for ingredients like niacinamide, hyaluronic acid, or ceramides that can hydrate your skin without making it feel greasy.

- **Treat:** If you have specific skin concerns like acne, blackheads, or hyperpigmentation, use targeted treatments like serums, spot treatments, or masks. Look for products with ingredients like salicylic acid, benzoyl peroxide, retinoids, or alpha hydroxy acids that can help unclog pores and exfoliate dead skin cells.

- **Apply Sunscreen:** Apply a broad-spectrum sunscreen with at least SPF 30 to protect your skin from harmful UV rays. Choose a product that's specifically formulated for oily skin and avoid any sunscreens that contain harsh chemicals like oxybenzone or avobenzone.

- **Use Blotting Papers:** Keep blotting papers with you to absorb any excess oil during the day without stripping away your skin's natural oils. Blotting papers can help to reduce shine and keep your skin looking fresh.

Good Skin Habits

- Cleansing your skin twice a day with a gentle cleanser formulated for oily skin.

- Using a toner that contains ingredients like salicylic acid, witch hazel, or tea tree oil helps control oil production and minimize pores.

- Moisturizing your skin daily with an oil-free moisturizer to keep it hydrated without adding excess oil.

- Exfoliating your skin once or twice a week with a gentle exfoliant to remove dead skin cells and unclog pores.

- Using products that contain ingredients like benzoyl peroxide, salicylic acid, or alpha-hydroxy acids helps control oil production and minimize breakouts.

- Using a broad-spectrum sunscreen with at least SPF 30 daily to protect your skin from harmful UV rays.

Bad Skin Habits

- Over washing your skin (it can strip away your skin's natural oils and cause it to produce even more oil)

- Using harsh or abrasive scrubs or exfoliants (they can damage your skin and cause irritation)

- Skipping moisturizing your skin (it can cause your skin to produce even more oil to compensate for the lack of moisture)

- Using products that contain heavy oils or pore-clogging ingredients like coconut oil, cocoa butter, or mineral oil.

- Touching your face too often (it can transfer bacteria and oils from your hands onto your skin)

- Using hot water to cleanse your skin (it can strip away your skin's natural oils and cause dryness)

Remember, the key to maintaining healthy skin is to balance the oil production in your skin without stripping it of its natural oils. Stick to a simple skincare routine with gentle, effective products, and avoid anything that can damage or irritate your skin.

Dry Skin

If you have dry skin, you know how uncomfortable it can be - the tightness, flakiness, and sometimes even itchiness. A consistent skincare regimen with the right products can help alleviate these symptoms and keep your skin hydrated and healthy. Here is a skincare regimen and some recommended products for dry skin:

- **Cleanser:** Use a gentle, non-foaming cleanser to avoid stripping your skin of its natural oils. Look for a creamy or oil-based cleanser that is free of harsh chemicals or fragrances.

- **Toner:** Use a hydrating toner to add an extra layer of moisture to your skin and help prepare it for other products. Look for a toner that contains humectants like glycerin or hyaluronic acid to attract and retain moisture.

- **Serum:** Use a hydrating serum to deliver concentrated moisture and nourishing ingredients to your skin. Look for a serum that contains hydrating ingredients like hyaluronic acid, ceramides, or glycerin.

- **Moisturizer:** Use a rich, emollient moisturizer to deeply hydrate your skin and protect it from moisture loss. Look for a moisturizer that contains nourishing ingredients like shea butter, squalane, or jojoba oil.

- **Sunscreen:** Use a broad-spectrum sunscreen with an SPF of at least 30 every day to protect your skin from the sun's harmful rays. Look for a sunscreen that is non-greasy and won't exacerbate your dryness.

- **Face Oil:** Using face oil as the last step in your routine can help lock in moisture and give your skin a healthy glow. Look for a face oil that is rich in nourishing ingredients like argan oil, marula oil, or rosehip oil.

Good Skin Habits

- Moisturizing your skin daily with a rich, hydrating moisturizer that contains ingredients like hyaluronic acid, ceramides, or glycerin to help lock in moisture.

- Using a gentle, non-foaming cleanser to avoid stripping away your skin's natural oils.

- Taking shorter, cooler showers to prevent further drying out your skin.

- Applying facial oil or serum containing vitamin E, C, or A to provide extra hydration.

- Using a humidifier in dry environments, such as your bedroom, to add moisture to the air and prevent your skin from drying out.

- Exfoliating your skin once a week with a gentle, hydrating exfoliant to remove dead skin cells and allow for better absorption of moisturizing products.

Bad Skin Habits

- Using hot water to wash your face or take a shower (it can further dry out your skin)

- Using harsh, fragranced, or alcohol-based products that can irritate and dry out your skin further.

- Over-exfoliating your skin (it can cause irritation and dryness)

- Using products with sulfates or other harsh detergents (they can strip your skin of its natural oils)

- Using hot air to dry your face or body (it can also dry out your skin)

- Using too many products or switching up your skincare routine too frequently (this can cause irritation and further dryness)

Remember, the key to caring for dry skin is to maintain the skin's natural moisture barrier and provide it with enough hydration to prevent further drying out. Stick to gentle, hydrating products, and avoid anything that can irritate or dry out your skin.

Combination skin

A skincare routine for combination skin should involve products that can address both oily and dry areas of the face. Here's a simple routine you can try:

- **Cleanse:** Start by washing your face with a gentle cleanser to remove dirt, oil, and makeup. Look for a cleanser that's specifically formulated for combination skin. You can use a foaming cleanser or a gel-based cleanser.

- **Tone:** After cleansing, use a toner to balance your skin's pH levels and remove any remaining impurities. Look for a toner that's alcohol-free, so it won't dry out your skin.

- **Treat:** If you have any specific skin concerns like acne, hyperpigmentation, or fine lines, you can apply a targeted treatment after toning. A serum with vitamin C, retinol, or hyaluronic acid can be beneficial for combination skin types.

- **Moisturize:** It's essential to moisturize both oily and dry areas of the face. Choose a lightweight moisturizer that won't clog your pores and still provide hydration to your skin. Look for ingredients like ceramides, glycerin, or hyaluronic acid, which can help retain moisture in your skin.

- **Apply Sunscreen:** Lastly, apply a broad-spectrum sunscreen with at least SPF 30 to protect your skin from harmful UV rays. This is especially important if you are using any active ingredients like retinol or AHAs, which can make your skin more sensitive to the sun.

Good Skin Habits

- Using a gentle, foaming cleanser to remove excess oil and impurities without drying out your skin.

- Using a toner that contains salicylic acid or witch hazel to help control oil production in your T-zone.

- Moisturizing your skin daily with a lightweight, oil-free moisturizer to hydrate your skin without adding excess oil.

- Using a broad-spectrum sunscreen with at least SPF 30 daily to protect your skin from harmful UV rays.

- Exfoliating your skin once or twice a week with a gentle exfoliant to remove dead skin cells and unclog pores.

- Using products that contain gentle ingredients like hyaluronic acid or glycerin to provide hydration to the dry areas of your skin.

Bad Skin Habits

- Over-washing your skin (it can strip away your skin's natural oils and cause it to produce even more oil)

- Using harsh or abrasive scrubs or exfoliants (they can damage your skin and cause irritation)

- Skipping moisturizing your skin (it can cause your skin to produce even more oil to compensate for the lack of moisture)

- Using heavy or pore-clogging products like thick creams or oils on your T-zone.

- Touching your face too often (it can transfer bacteria and oils from your hands onto your skin)

- Using hot water to cleanse your skin (it can strip away your skin's natural oils and cause dryness)

Remember, combination skin requires a balancing act of hydrating dry areas while controlling excess oil production in the T-zone. Stick to a simple skincare routine with gentle, effective products and avoid anything that can damage or irritate your skin.

Sensitive Skin

When it comes to a skincare routine for sensitive skin, it's important to choose gentle and non-irritating products that won't cause any redness, itching, or inflammation. Here's a simple routine you can try:

- **Cleanse:** Start by washing your face with a gentle, fragrance-free cleanser that won't strip your skin's natural oils. Look for a product that's specifically formulated for sensitive skin.

- **Tone:** After cleansing, use a gentle toner that's alcohol-free and contains soothing ingredients like chamomile, aloe vera, or green tea extract. This can help to calm any redness or irritation and restore your skin's pH balance.

- **Moisturize:** Apply a lightweight, fragrance-free moisturizer that's suitable for sensitive skin. Look for ingredients like ceramides, hyaluronic acid, or shea butter, which can provide hydration and nourishment to your skin.

- **Apply Sunscreen:** Apply a broad-spectrum sunscreen with at least SPF 30 to protect your skin from harmful UV rays. Choose a product that's specifically formulated for sensitive skin and avoid any sunscreens that contain harsh chemicals like oxybenzone or avobenzone.

- **Avoid Harsh Products:** It's important to avoid using any harsh or abrasive products like scrubs, exfoliants, or peels. These can irritate sensitive skin and cause redness, itching, or inflammation.

- **Patch-Test New Products:** Whenever you introduce a new skincare product, it's important to patch-test it first. Apply a small amount of the product on your inner arm or behind your ear and wait for twenty-four hours to see if you have any allergic reactions.

Remember, less is more when it comes to skincare for sensitive skin. Stick to a simple routine with gentle, fragrance-free products, and avoid anything that can cause irritation or inflammation.

Good Skin Habits

- Using gentle, fragrance-free, and non-irritating skincare products specifically formulated for sensitive skin.

- Patch testing new products on a small area of your skin before using them on your entire face.

- Moisturizing your skin regularly with a gentle, hydrating moisturizer to help soothe and protect your skin.

- Using a broad-spectrum sunscreen with at least SPF 30 daily to protect your skin from harmful UV rays.

- Using lukewarm water to cleanse your skin

- Applying a cool compress or use aloe vera gel to soothe any redness, irritation, or inflammation.

Bad Skin Habits

- Using harsh scrubs or exfoliants (they can irritate and damage your skin)

- Using products with fragrances, alcohol, or other potential irritants.

- Using hot water to wash your face (it can cause further irritation and dryness)

- Over-exfoliating your skin (it can lead to irritation and sensitivity)

- Using products with abrasive or harsh ingredients, such as retinoids or alpha-hydroxy acids.

- Using too many products or switching up your skincare routine too frequently (this can cause irritation and further sensitivity)

Remember, sensitive skin requires extra care and attention to avoid irritation and inflammation. Use gentle, non-irritating products, avoid harsh or abrasive ingredients, and be consistent with your skincare routine to keep your skin calm and healthy.

SECTION NINE

Skincare and Makeup

SECTION NINE

Skincare and Makeup

The Flawless Fusion

Skincare and makeup are two inseparable aspects of beauty routines, and it is not hard to see why. While skincare focuses on nourishing and taking care of your skin, makeup is a way to enhance your natural features and create a flawless look. These two beauty categories often overlap, with the application of makeup often influencing skincare and vice versa.

Skincare and Makeup Intersection

Skincare and makeup may seem like completely different beauty categories, but they share common ground when it comes to ingredients, benefits, and application techniques. For example, many skincare products contain ingredients that also appear in makeup, such as hyaluronic acid and vitamin C. These ingredients have been shown to help hydrate and brighten the skin, which is essential for a smooth makeup application.

Similarly, makeup can benefit your skincare routine by protecting your skin from the sun and environmental damage. Many makeup products, such as tinted moisturizers and foundations, now include broad-spectrum SPF protection, which can help prevent sun damage and premature aging. Additionally, makeup can act as a barrier between your skin and pollutants, dust, and other environmental irritants.

Finally, the application of makeup can also influence skincare routines. For example, using a gentle cleanser to remove makeup can help prevent breakouts and irritation, while applying a hydrating serum or moisturizer before makeup application can create a smooth base for foundation and other makeup products.

Makeup and Skincare Benefits

Skincare and makeup both offer a range of benefits that can improve the overall health and appearance of your skin. Skincare products are designed to hydrate, protect, and nourish your skin, while makeup products can help enhance your natural features, even out your skin tone, and create a flawless, polished look.

Some of the specific benefits of skincare products include:

- **Hydration:** Many skincare products, such as moisturizers and serums, are designed to hydrate and nourish the skin, helping to keep it looking healthy and youthful.

- **Protection:** Skincare products can also help protect your skin from environmental damage, such as pollution and UV rays, which can cause premature aging and other skin issues.

- **Anti-Aging:** Many skincare products are formulated with ingredients that can help reduce the appearance of fine lines, wrinkles, and other signs of aging.

Meanwhile, some of the specific benefits of makeup products include:

- **Even Skin Tone:** Makeup products, such as foundation and concealer, can help even out your skin tone and cover up imperfections, such as blemishes, redness, and dark circles.

- **Enhancing Natural Features:** Makeup products, such as mascara and lipstick, can help enhance your natural looks and add a pop of color to your skin.

- **Boosting Confidence:** Finally, makeup can also help boost your confidence and make you feel more put-together and polished.

Choosing the Right Makeup Products

Foundation: Finding the Perfect Match

Foundation serves as the base for your makeup look, providing coverage and creating a smooth canvas. Choosing the right foundation is crucial to achieving a natural and flawless finish. As a dermatologist, we understand the importance of selecting a foundation that not only matches your skin tone but also caters to your skin type.

When choosing a foundation, consider the following factors:

- **Skin Tone:** Determine your undertone—whether it's warm, cool, or neutral—to find a foundation shade that complements your complexion. Test the foundation on your jawline or the back of your hand to ensure it blends seamlessly with your skin.

- **Coverage:** Assess the level of coverage you desire. Sheer or light coverage foundations provide a more natural and dewy look, while medium to full coverage foundations offer more concealment for blemishes or discoloration.

- **Skin Type:** Consider your skin type when selecting a foundation formula. If you have oily skin, opt for oil-free or matte foundations that help control shine. Dry skin benefits from hydrating foundations with moisturizing ingredients. Combination skin may require a balanced formula that addresses both oily and dry areas.

- **Finish:** Decide on the finish you prefer. Matte foundations provide a shine-free look, ideal for oily or combination skin. Dewy or luminous foundations give a radiant glow, perfect for dry or dull skin. Satin or natural finishes offer a balance between matte and dewy, suitable for various skin types.

Remember, it's essential to test the foundation on your skin before purchasing it. Many beauty stores offer samples or testers, allowing you to try different shades and formulas. Also, take into account any specific skin concerns or sensitivities you may have and choose foundations labeled as non-comedogenic or hypoallergenic for a lower risk of irritation or breakouts.

Concealer: Camouflaging Imperfections

Concealers are like magic wands, helping to hide imperfections such as dark circles, blemishes, or redness. They offer additional coverage where needed, creating a more even complexion. To choose the right concealer, consider the following:

- **Shade:** Select a concealer shade that closely matches your foundation or is slightly lighter to brighten the under-eye area. Avoid going too dark, as it may accentuate rather than conceal imperfections.

- **Formulation:** Concealers come in various formulations, including liquids, creams, sticks, and pens. Liquid concealers offer lightweight coverage and work well for the under-eye area. Cream concealers provide more coverage for blemishes or discoloration. Choose a formulation that suits your preferences and the specific area you want to conceal.

- **Texture:** Consider the texture of the concealer based on your skin type. Creamy concealers are suitable for dry skin, while matte or oil-free options work better for oily skin. Blendability is also important to ensure a seamless application.

- **Application Technique:** Explore different application techniques, such as using a brush, sponge, or fingers, to find the method that gives you the desired coverage and finish. Patting or dabbing motions help blend the concealer effectively.

Remember to set the concealer with a light dusting of translucent powder to enhance its longevity and prevent creasing.

Blush and Bronzer: Adding Color and Definition

Blush and bronzer add a touch of color, warmth, and dimension to the face. They can bring life to your complexion and accentuate your features. Here's what you should consider when selecting blush and bronzer:

- **Skin Tone:** Choose blush shades that complement your skin tone. Rosy pinks and peachy tones work well for fair to light skin tones, while deeper berry or coral shades suit medium to dark skin tones. For bronzer, select shades that mimic a natural sun-kissed glow. Opt for warmer, golden tones for fair to medium skin tones, and deeper, richer shades for darker skin tones.

- **Formulation:** Blush and bronzer come in different formulations, including powders, creams, and liquids. Powder blushes and bronzers are versatile and easy to blend, making them a popular choice for most skin types. Cream or liquid formulas can provide a dewier and more natural finish, ideal for those with dry skin.

- **Finish:** Consider the desired finish for your blush and bronzer. Matte formulations offer a soft, natural look, while shimmer or satin finishes add a touch of radiance and glow.

Choose a finish that complements your overall makeup look and personal style.

- **Application Technique:** Use a fluffy brush for powder blush and bronzer application, tapping off any excess product before applying. Apply blush on the apples of your cheeks and blend it towards the temples for a natural flush. For bronzer, lightly dust it on areas where the sun naturally hits the face, such as the forehead, cheekbones, and jawline, to create a sun-kissed effect.

Remember to start with a light hand and build up the color gradually for a more natural and blended result. Blending is key to achieving a seamless and flattering application.

Eye Makeup: Enhancing Your Eyes

Eye makeup has the power to transform and enhance the eyes, adding depth, definition, and drama. When selecting eye makeup products, consider the following:

- **Eyeshadow:** Choose eyeshadow colors that complement your eye color and skin tone. Neutrals, such as browns and taupes, are versatile options that work for most occasions. Experiment with different finishes, including matte, shimmer, and metallic, to create various looks. Consider eyeshadow palettes that offer a range of colors for versatility.

- **Eyeliner:** Decide on the type of eyeliner that suits your preferences and skill level. Pencil eyeliners are beginner-friendly and can create both subtle and bold looks. Liquid eyeliners offer precise and sharp lines, ideal for creating winged or cat-eye looks. Gel or cream eyeliners provide long-lasting wear and are perfect for smudged or smoky effects.

- **Mascara:** Look for mascaras that provide volume, length, or both, depending on your desired effect. Consider the formula, brush shape, and whether you prefer waterproof or non-waterproof options. Mascara can help define and accentuate your lashes, opening up your eyes.

- **Eyebrows:** Enhancing your eyebrows can frame your face and complete your eye makeup look. Choose eyebrow products, such as pencils, powders, or gels, that match your eyebrow color and allow for precise application. Fill in sparse areas and shape your brows to achieve a polished appearance.

Experiment with different eye makeup techniques, such as smokey eyes, cut creases, or natural everyday looks, to find what suits your style and occasion. Don't forget to use eyeshadow primers to improve longevity and prevent creasing.

Lip Products: Creating a Luscious Pout

Lip products can add a finishing touch to your makeup look, whether you desire a bold statement or a subtle enhancement. Consider the following when choosing lip products:

- **Lipstick:** Lipsticks come in various shades, finishes, and formulations. Select colors that complement your skin tone and match your desired look. Nude shades, pinks, reds, and berry tones are popular choices. Matte lipsticks offer a long-lasting and velvety finish, while satin or creamy formulas provide hydration and a lustrous sheen.

- **Lip Gloss:** Lip glosses add shine and dimension to the lips, creating a youthful and plump appearance. They come in clear or tinted formulations, offering a range of finishes from sheer to high-shine. Choose a lip gloss that complements your lip color or wear it alone for a natural, glossy look.

- **Lip Liner:** Lip liners help define and shape the lips, prevent feathering or bleeding of lip products, and prolong their wear. Select a lip liner that matches your natural lip color or the shade of lipstick or gloss you plan to wear. Outline the lips and fill them in for a more long-lasting and defined result.

- **Lip Balm:** Lip balm is an essential product for maintaining hydrated and healthy lips. Look for lip balms with moisturizing ingredients like shea butter, coconut oil, or hyaluronic acid. Use lip balm regularly to keep your lips smooth, soft, and primed for lip product application.

Consider your personal style, occasion, and comfort level when choosing lip products. Experiment with different colors and finishes to find the ones that make you feel confident and beautiful.

Remember, proper lip care is essential. Exfoliate your lips gently with a lip scrub or a soft toothbrush to remove dry skin before applying lip products. Additionally, stay hydrated by drinking plenty of water to keep your lips and skin hydrated from within.

By selecting the right makeup products for your foundation, concealer, blush and bronzer, eye makeup, and lip products, you can create a personalized and beautiful makeup look. Don't forget to consider your skin type, skin tone, and desired finish to achieve the best results. Experiment, have fun, and embrace the transformative power of makeup while caring for your skin's health and well-being.

Makeup Application Techniques

Foundation Application: Achieving Flawless Coverage

Applying foundation properly is the key to achieving a smooth and flawless complexion. Follow these steps for a seamless foundation application:

- **Step 1:** Prep your skin by cleansing and moisturizing it. Allow the moisturizer to fully absorb before moving on to the next step.

- **Step 2:** Choose a foundation that matches your skin tone and type. Use a foundation brush, makeup sponge, or clean fingertips for application.

- **Step 3:** Start by applying small dots of foundation to your forehead, cheeks, nose, and chin. This helps distribute the product evenly.

- **Step 4:** Blend the foundation using gentle outward strokes, focusing on areas that require more coverage, such as redness or blemishes. Blend carefully along the jawline and hairline to avoid any noticeable lines.

- **Step 5:** If needed, build up the coverage by applying an additional thin layer of foundation only to the areas that require more attention.

- **Step 6:** Set the foundation with a light dusting of translucent powder to prolong its wear and reduce shine.

Concealer Techniques: Correcting and Highlighting

Concealer is a versatile product that helps camouflage imperfections and brighten specific areas of the face. Here's how to use concealer effectively:

- **Step 1:** After applying foundation, choose a concealer that matches your skin tone or is slightly lighter for under-eye brightening.

- **Step 2:** Use a small, precise brush or a makeup sponge to apply concealer directly to areas of concern, such as under-eye circles, blemishes, or redness.

- **Step 3:** Gently blend the concealer using tapping or patting motions with your fingertips or a sponge. Avoid rubbing or dragging the product, as it can disrupt the coverage.

- **Step 4:** To brighten the under-eye area, apply concealer in an upside-down triangle shape, extending from the inner corner of the eye to the outer corner and blending it seamlessly with the surrounding skin.

- **Step 5:** Set the concealer by lightly dusting a translucent or setting powder over the areas where you applied concealer.

Eye Makeup Application: From Basic to Glamorous

Enhancing your eyes with makeup can make a significant difference in your overall look. Follow these steps for eye makeup application:

- **Step 1:** Start by applying an eyeshadow primer to create a smooth base and prolong the wear of your eye makeup.

- **Step 2:** Choose eyeshadow shades that complement your eye color and the desired look. Begin with a neutral or transition shade to define the crease.

- **Step 3:** Apply a medium-tone shade on the eyelid, blending it softly into the crease color for a seamless transition.

- **Step 4:** Use a darker shade or eyeliner along the upper lash line to add definition. Blend it well for a smudged or smoky effect.

- **Step 5:** Apply a lighter eyeshadow shade or shimmer on the inner corners of the eyes and under the brow bone to create a highlight.

- **Step 6:** Curl your lashes with an eyelash curler and apply mascara to add volume and length. Wiggle the wand at the roots and sweep it upward for maximum effect.

- **Step 7:** For a more glamorous look, consider adding false lashes or experimenting with eyeliner styles like winged or cat-eye.

Blush and Bronzer Application: Sculpting Your Features

Blush and bronzer add dimension and definition to the face. Follow these steps for a natural and sculpted look:

- **Step 1:** Smile to identify the apples of your cheeks, where the blush should be applied.

- **Step 2:** Using a blush brush, pick up a small amount of blush and tap off any excess product.

- **Step 3:** Gently sweep the blush onto the apples of your cheeks in a soft, upward motion toward your temples. Blend the color well to create a natural flush.

- **Step 4:** To add warmth and contour to your face, use a bronzer. Choose a shade that complements your skin tone and mimics a sun-kissed glow.

- **Step 5:** Using a fluffy brush, lightly dust the bronzer onto areas where the sun naturally hits, such as the forehead, cheekbones, and jawline. Blend it well to create a subtle, bronzed effect.

- **Step 6:** If desired, you can also contour your face by applying a slightly deeper shade of bronzer in the hollows of your cheeks, along the jawline, and on the sides of your nose. Blend it carefully for a natural-looking sculpted effect.

Lip Makeup Application: Creating Beautiful Lips

Lip makeup can enhance your smile and complete your overall look. Follow these steps for a polished and beautiful lip application:

- **Step 1:** Start by exfoliating your lips to remove any dry or flaky skin. You can use a lip scrub or gently massage your lips with a soft toothbrush.

- **Step 2:** Apply a lip balm to moisturize and prep your lips for color. Allow it to absorb for a few minutes before moving on to the next step.

- **Step 3:** Choose a lip liner that matches your natural lip color or the shade of lipstick you'll be using. Begin by outlining the natural shape of your lips to define their contours.

- **Step 4:** Fill in your lips with the lip liner to create a base that helps the lipstick last longer and prevents feathering.

- **Step 5:** Select a lipstick shade that complements your skin tone and the desired look. Apply the lipstick directly from the tube or use a lip brush for more precise application.

- **Step 6:** Blot your lips gently with a tissue to remove any excess product and create a long-lasting finish.

- **Step 7:** For added shine and dimension, you can apply a lip gloss to the center of your lips. This creates a fuller and more luscious appearance.

Remember to experiment with different colors, textures, and finishes to find the lip makeup that suits your personal style and the occasion. With practice, you'll become more confident in your makeup application techniques, allowing you to create beautiful and customized looks for any situation.

Removing makeup and post-makeup skincare

Importance of Makeup Removal

Once you have understood makeup application, it's crucial to understand the importance of makeup removal. Leaving makeup on overnight can have negative effects on your skin's health and appearance. Here's why makeup removal is essential:

- **Skin Health:** Makeup, especially foundation and concealer, can clog your pores, leading to breakouts, blackheads, and acne. Proper removal allows your skin to breathe and prevents the buildup of impurities.

- **Skin Renewal:** During sleep, your skin goes through a process of rejuvenation and repair. Leaving makeup on hinders this process, as it can interfere with the natural exfoliation and cell turnover. Removing makeup allows your skin to renew itself effectively.

- **Preventing Irritation:** Some makeup products contain ingredients that can irritate the skin, causing redness, itching, or inflammation. By thoroughly removing makeup, you minimize the risk of irritation and sensitivity.

- **Eye Health:** Mascara, eyeliner, and eyeshadow can cause irritation and potential infections if left on the eyes for an extended period. Removing eye makeup gently helps maintain eye health and prevents issues, such as styes or dryness.

Makeup Removal Techniques: Cleansing, Toning, and Moisturizing

To ensure proper makeup removal and maintain healthy skin, follow these essential steps:

- **Step 1:** Start by selecting a gentle and suitable makeup remover based on your skin type. Options include micellar water, cleansing balms, oils, or makeup remover wipes.

- **Step 2:** Begin with the eyes. Soak a cotton pad or a clean cloth with the makeup remover and gently press it against closed eyelids. Hold for a few seconds to allow the product to dissolve the eye makeup, and then gently wipe away the makeup, moving from the inner to the outer corner of the eye. Be careful not to tug or rub too harshly.

- **Step 3:** Move on to the face. Take a small amount of makeup remover on your fingertips or a cotton pad and apply it to the face, focusing on areas with heavy makeup or stubborn residue.

Massage the remover into the skin in gentle circular motions, ensuring thorough coverage.

- **Step 4:** Rinse your face with lukewarm water to remove the makeup remover and any remaining traces of makeup. Pat your face dry with a clean towel.

- **Step 5:** Follow up with a gentle facial cleanser appropriate for your skin type. Massage the cleanser onto damp skin, focusing on the areas where makeup was applied. Rinse thoroughly with water and pat dry.

- **Step 6:** After cleansing, apply a toner suitable for your skin type. Toners help remove any residual impurities, balance the skin's pH, and prepare it for the next skincare steps.

- **Step 7:** Finish by applying a moisturizer or night cream to hydrate and nourish your skin. Choose a moisturizer that suits your skin's needs, whether it is oil-free for oily skin, hydrating for dry skin, or anti-aging for mature skin.

Post-Makeup Skincare: Restoring and Nourishing the Skin

After makeup removal, it is essential to give your skin some extra care and attention. Consider the following post-makeup skincare steps to restore and nourish your skin:

- **Exfoliation:** Regular exfoliation helps remove dead skin cells and promotes a fresh and radiant complexion. Use a gentle exfoliating scrub or a chemical exfoliant suitable for your skin type, and follow the instructions provided.

- **Face Masks:** Choose a face mask that caters to your skin's needs. For dry skin, opt for a moisturizing mask with ingredients like hyaluronic acid or aloe vera. If you have oily or acne-prone skin, look for masks containing ingredients like clay or salicylic acid to help control excess oil and minimize breakouts. Apply the mask to clean the skin, leave it on for the recommended time, and then rinse it off thoroughly.

- **Serums and Treatments:** Incorporate targeted serums or treatments into your skincare routine to address specific concerns. Whether it's brightening, anti-aging, or acne-fighting, serums packed with active ingredients can provide an extra boost to your skin. Apply a few drops of serum to your face and gently massage it in, focusing on areas that need attention.

- **Eye Cream:** The delicate skin around the eyes requires special care. Apply a nourishing eye cream or gel to help hydrate, reduce puffiness, and diminish the appearance of fine lines and dark circles. Use your ring finger to gently pat the product around the eye area, avoiding any harsh rubbing or pulling.

- **Moisturize:** Finish your skincare routine by applying a moisturizer suitable for your skin type. Moisturizers help hydrate, nourish, and protect the skin. Choose a lightweight formula for oily skin or a richer cream for dry skin. Apply the moisturizer evenly to your face and neck, using upward and outward motions.

- **Sun Protection:** Don't forget the importance of sunscreen, even if you're not wearing makeup. Apply a broad-spectrum sunscreen with an SPF of 30 or higher as the final step in your skincare routine. Sunscreen helps protect your skin from harmful UV rays, preventing premature aging, sun damage, and skin discoloration.

Makeup and Skincare for Different Skin Types

Everyone's skin is unique, and understanding your specific skin type is crucial for selecting the right makeup and skincare products. In this section, we will explore the special considerations and recommendations for different skin types:

Oily Skin

If you have oily skin, you may struggle with excess sebum production and a shiny complexion. Here are some tips for managing oily skin with makeup and skincare:

- Look for oil-free and mattifying foundation and powder formulas that help control shine throughout the day.
- Use blotting papers or oil-absorbing sheets to remove excess oil without disturbing your makeup.
- Choose lightweight, water-based moisturizers and gel-based cleansers that won't clog your pores.
- Opt for oil-free or non-comedogenic products to prevent breakouts.
- Consider using a mattifying primer before applying makeup to create a smooth canvas and prolong the wear of your foundation.

Dry Skin

If your skin tends to be dry and lacks moisture, it requires extra hydration and nourishment. Consider the following recommendations:

- Use a rich, hydrating foundation or tinted moisturizer to add moisture and create a dewy complexion.
- Prioritize skincare products with hydrating ingredients like hyaluronic acid, glycerin, and ceramides.
- Avoid matte or powder-based products that can accentuate dryness and fine lines.
- Look for creamy or liquid blushes and bronzers that add a healthy glow to your skin.

- Incorporate a nourishing facial oil or moisturizing mask into your skincare routine to provide intense hydration.

Combination Skin

- Combination skin can be a mix of oily and dry areas, requiring a balanced approach. Here's what you need to know:
- Use a lightweight, oil-free foundation or BB cream to provide coverage without overwhelming oily areas.
- Consider spot-concealing only where necessary instead of applying heavy foundation all over your face.
- Use a gentle cleanser that cleanses without stripping the skin's natural oils.
- Consider using a toner to balance the skin's pH levels and minimize excess oil production.
- Apply a lightweight moisturizer on dry areas and avoid heavy creams on oily zones.

Sensitive Skin

Sensitive skin can be easily irritated and may react to certain ingredients. Here are some recommendations for makeup and skincare:

- Opt for fragrance-free and hypoallergenic products to minimize the risk of irritation.
- Perform patch tests on new products before applying them to your face.
- Choose gentle cleansers and makeup removers that don't disrupt the skin's natural barrier.
- Look for skincare products with soothing ingredients like aloe vera, chamomile, or oatmeal.
- Avoid harsh exfoliants and opt for gentle, chemical exfoliants if necessary.

Makeup and Skincare for Mature Skin

As we age, our skin goes through changes, such as loss of elasticity and the appearance of fine lines and wrinkles. Consider the following tips for makeup and skincare for mature skin:

Anti-Aging Makeup

- Choose a lightweight foundation with a luminous or satin finish to avoid emphasizing wrinkles and fine lines.

- Use a creamy concealer to brighten the under-eye area and conceal any discoloration.

- Avoid heavy powders that can settle into fine lines and make the skin look dry.

- Opt for cream blushes and bronzers to add a youthful, natural flush of color to the cheeks.

- Consider using a luminizing highlighter to bring a subtle glow to areas like the cheekbones and brow bones.

Skincare for Mature Skin

- Incorporate anti-aging ingredients like retinol, peptides, and antioxidants into your skincare routine to help address the specific concerns of mature skin.

- Use a gentle cleanser that doesn't strip the skin of its natural oils and opt for hydrating or nourishing formulas.

- Apply a moisturizer with rich texture to provide intense hydration and support the skin's natural barrier function.

- Incorporate serums or creams with ingredients like hyaluronic acid, vitamin C, or niacinamide to target fine lines, wrinkles, and uneven skin tone.

- Don't forget to include an eye cream specifically formulated for mature skin to address concerns such as crow's feet and sagging eyelids.

- Consider using a facial oil as a final step to lock in moisture and provide additional nourishment to the skin.

- Protect your skin from the sun by using a broad-spectrum sunscreen with a high SPF rating. This helps prevent further damage and minimize the appearance of sunspots and wrinkles.

Dealing with Common Makeup and Skincare Challenges

Acne-Prone Skin

- Choose non-comedogenic, oil-free, and lightweight makeup products that won't clog your pores.

- Cleanse your skin thoroughly and avoid using heavy, occlusive products that can trap bacteria and cause breakouts.

- Use spot treatments with ingredients like benzoyl peroxide or salicylic acid to target blemishes.

- Be cautious with makeup brushes and sponges, as they can harbor bacteria. Clean them regularly to prevent the spread of acne-causing bacteria.

Hyperpigmentation

- Use color-correcting products with green or peach undertones to neutralize and balance out discoloration.

- Choose foundations and concealers that provide buildable coverage to camouflage hyperpigmentation without looking heavy or cakey.

- Incorporate skincare products with brightening ingredients like vitamin C, kojic acid, or licorice extract to help fade dark spots over time.

- Protect your skin from the sun by wearing sunscreen daily to prevent further darkening of hyperpigmented areas.

Under-Eye Circles

- Use color correctors with peach or orange undertones to neutralize dark circles before applying concealer.

- Opt for lightweight, hydrating concealers that brighten the under-eye area without settling into fine lines.

- Apply eye creams with ingredients like caffeine or hyaluronic acid to help reduce puffiness and hydrate the delicate skin around the eyes.

- Use a gentle tapping motion with your ring finger to apply concealer and avoid pulling or tugging on the delicate skin.

Redness and Rosacea

- Use green-tinted primers or color-correcting creams to neutralize redness before applying foundation.

- Choose foundations with buildable coverage and a yellow undertone to counteract redness.

- Avoid products with irritants like fragrance or alcohol, which can aggravate redness and sensitivity.

- Incorporate skincare products with calming ingredients like chamomile or aloe vera to soothe redness and inflammation.

Makeup and Skincare for Special Occasions

For special occasions, you may want to enhance your makeup and skincare routine to achieve a specific look or long-lasting wear. Here are some considerations:

Bridal and Wedding Makeup

- Invest in a high-quality, long-wearing foundation and concealer to withstand tears, sweat, and long hours.

- Use a primer to create a smooth base and ensure your makeup lasts throughout the day.

- Consider using waterproof or smudge-proof products, especially for mascara and eyeliner.

- Opt for a setting spray to lock your makeup in place and help it withstand the

- test of time.

- Choose a lip color that complements your overall look and lasts through the day. Consider using a lip primer and a long-wearing lipstick or lip stain.

- Don't forget to touch up your makeup throughout the day or have a trusted friend or professional on hand for any necessary touch-ups.

Evening and Party Makeup

- Experiment with bolder and more dramatic looks, such as smoky eyes or vibrant eyeshadow colors.

- Use eyeliners and mascaras that offer intense pigmentation and long-lasting wear.

- Consider using false lashes or lash extensions to enhance your eye makeup.

- Choose long-wearing and transfer-resistant lip products to avoid constant reapplication.

- Incorporate highlighting products to add a radiant glow to your complexion for evening events.

Seasonal and Holiday Looks

- Embrace seasonal trends and colors in your makeup choices, such as warm tones for autumn or metallic shades for the holidays.

- Adjust your skincare routine to address seasonal changes, like using a heavier moisturizer in winter or incorporating a hydrating mask for dry summer months.

- Protect your skin from harsh weather conditions, such as using a moisturizing lip balm in cold weather or applying sunscreen during sunny outdoor events.

- Consider using setting sprays or powders to prolong the wear of your makeup, especially during long holiday celebrations

Makeup is an essential part of many people's daily beauty routines. While makeup can help enhance your natural features and boost your confidence, it's essential to use it properly to avoid potential skin problems and other issues. Let us conclude this section by mentioning some habits related to makeup and skincare:

Good Skin Habits

- Always start with a clean, moisturized face: Before applying makeup, make sure your skin is clean and moisturized. This will create a smooth base for your makeup and help it last longer.

- Use makeup brushes and sponges: Use makeup brushes and sponges to apply your makeup, as using your fingers can transfer oils and bacteria to your face.

- Choose makeup that is appropriate for your skin type: Choose makeup products that are appropriate for your skin type, whether you have oily, dry, or sensitive skin.

- Use a primer: Apply a primer to your face before applying your makeup. This will help your makeup go on more smoothly and stay in place throughout the day.

- Remove your makeup before bed: Always remove your makeup before bed, as leaving it on overnight can clog your pores and lead to breakouts.

Bad Skin Habits

- Sharing makeup: Sharing makeup with others can transfer bacteria and lead to infections.

- Sleeping with makeup on: Leaving makeup on overnight can clog your pores and lead to breakouts.

- Using expired makeup: Expired makeup can harbor bacteria and lead to skin irritation and infections.

- Overdoing it: Avoid using too much makeup, as this can look unnatural and caked-on. Instead, use a light hand and build up your coverage gradually.

- Forgetting to clean your makeup tools: Dirty makeup tools can harbor bacteria and lead to skin problems. Clean your brushes and sponges regularly with gentle soap and water or a specialized makeup brush cleaner.

Makeup can be a fun and effective way to enhance your natural beauty, but it's essential to use it properly to avoid skin problems and other issues. By choosing good habits for makeup, you can help ensure that your makeup looks great and is healthy for your skin.

SECTION TEN

Skin Supplements!

SECTION TEN

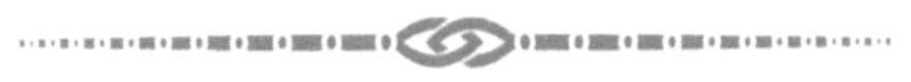

Skin Supplements!

Your Skin Shows What You Eat!

Our skin is the most visible organ of our body, and what we eat can have a significant impact on its health and appearance. Just as certain foods can help nourish and protect the skin, others can damage it and accelerate the aging process. In recent years, the use of oral skin supplements has become increasingly popular. In the previous sections we have discussed the good foods for skin, here we will shed some light on the various skin supplements available in the market, and their role in our skin health.

Skin supplements are oral dietary supplements that contain specific nutrients and ingredients aimed at improving skin health and addressing various skin concerns. These supplements work from within, nourishing the body with essential nutrients that support the structure, function, and overall well-being of the skin

There are many different types of oral skin supplements available on the market, and each one contains a unique blend of ingredients that are designed to provide specific benefits to the skin. Some of the most common ingredients found in these supplements include collagen, hyaluronic acid, vitamins A, C, and E, and various antioxidants.

Collagen

Collagen is a protein that is naturally found in the body and is essential for maintaining healthy skin. As we age, our bodies produce less collagen, which can lead to the formation of wrinkles and fine lines. Collagen supplements are designed to provide the body with the necessary building blocks to produce more collagen, which can help to improve skin elasticity and reduce the appearance of fine lines and wrinkles.

Hyaluronic Acid

Hyaluronic acid is a substance that is naturally found in the body and is essential for maintaining hydrated and healthy skin. This substance is responsible for keeping the skin plump and hydrated, and as we age, our bodies produce less of it. Hyaluronic acid supplements are designed to provide the body with this essential substance, which can help to improve skin hydration and reduce the appearance of fine lines and wrinkles.

Vitamin A

Vitamin A, also known as retinol, is a powerful antioxidant that promotes healthy skin cell turnover. It aids in the production of collagen and elastin, which contribute to skin elasticity and firmness. Vitamin A also helps reduce the appearance of fine lines, wrinkles, and hyperpigmentation.

Vitamin C

Vitamin C is a vital nutrient for collagen synthesis, a protein that provides structure to the skin. It helps protect the skin against oxidative stress, aids in wound healing, and brightens the complexion. Vitamin C also has antioxidant properties, which neutralize free radicals and help prevent skin damage caused by environmental factors.

Vitamin E

Vitamin E is a potent antioxidant that helps protect the skin against free radicals, which can accelerate the aging process and lead to skin damage. It supports skin hydration, reduces inflammation, and promotes wound healing. Vitamin E works synergistically with other antioxidants, such as vitamin C, to enhance their effectiveness.

Vitamin B Complex

B vitamins, including Biotin (B7), Niacin (B3), and Riboflavin (B2), play a vital role in maintaining healthy skin. Biotin supports the production of keratin, a protein that contributes to healthy hair, skin, and nails. Niacin helps improve skin barrier function and reduce redness, while Riboflavin enhances cellular energy production, promoting a radiant complexion.

Vitamin D

This vitamin is important for maintaining healthy bones and may also have benefits for skin health. Vitamin D supplements are thought to help improve skin texture and reduce the risk of skin cancer.

Coenzyme Q10 (CoQ10)

This antioxidant is naturally produced by the body and is involved in the production of energy in cells. CoQ10 supplements are thought to help reduce the appearance of fine lines and wrinkles and improve skin texture.

Omega-3 Fatty Acids

These essential fatty acids are important for maintaining healthy skin and can be found in foods like fatty fish, flaxseed, and chia seeds. Omega-3 supplements are thought to help reduce inflammation in the body and improve skin hydration.

Probiotics

These beneficial bacteria can help improve gut health, which in turn can lead to improvements in skin health. Probiotic supplements are thought to help reduce inflammation in the body and improve the appearance of acne-prone skin.

Zinc

This mineral is important for maintaining healthy skin and can be found in foods like oysters, beef, and pumpkin seeds. Zinc supplements are thought to help reduce inflammation in the body and improve the appearance of acne-prone skin.

Ceramides

These naturally occurring lipids help to keep the skin hydrated and protected. Ceramide supplements are thought to help improve skin hydration and reduce the appearance of fine lines and wrinkles.

Resveratrol

This antioxidant is found in grapes and red wine and has been shown to have anti-inflammatory and anti-aging properties. Resveratrol supplements are thought to help improve skin texture and reduce the appearance of fine lines and wrinkles.

Lycopene

This antioxidant is found in tomatoes and has been shown to have photoprotective properties. Lycopene supplements are thought to help protect the skin from sun damage and improve skin hydration.

Polypodium Leucotomos Extract

This extract comes from a fern plant and has been shown to have photoprotective properties. Polypodium leucotomos extract supplements are thought to help protect the skin from sun damage and reduce the risk of skin cancer.

Glutathione

This antioxidant is naturally produced by the body and is involved in the detoxification process. Glutathione supplements are thought to help reduce inflammation in the body and improve skin health.

Skin Concerns and Supplements

Acne-Prone Skin

Acne is a common skin concern characterized by the formation of pimples, blackheads, and whiteheads. Several supplements can help manage acne-prone skin. Zinc supplements can help regulate oil production, reduce inflammation, and support skin healing. Vitamin A, in the form of retinoids or beta-carotene, promotes skin cell turnover and regulates sebum production. Omega-3 fatty acids have anti-inflammatory properties that can help reduce acne-related inflammation and improve overall skin health.

Aging Skin

As we age, our skin experiences a natural decline in collagen production, leading to the appearance of fine lines, wrinkles, and sagging skin. To address aging skin concerns, collagen peptides can be taken as supplements to support the body's collagen synthesis and improve skin elasticity. Resveratrol, a powerful antioxidant found in grapes and berries, helps protect the skin from oxidative stress and may have anti-aging effects. Coenzyme Q10, naturally present in the body, supports cellular energy production and helps reduce the signs of aging.

Dry and Dehydrated Skin

Dry and dehydrated skin lacks moisture and often feels tight and rough. Hyaluronic acid supplements can help replenish moisture levels in the skin by attracting and retaining water, resulting in improved hydration and a plumper complexion. Omega-3 fatty acids, particularly EPA and DHA, nourish the skin from within, supporting the skin's natural oil barrier and preventing moisture loss, leading to smoother and suppler skin.

Hyperpigmentation

Hyperpigmentation refers to areas of the skin that have darkened due to increased melanin production. Vitamin C supplements can help brighten the skin and reduce the appearance of hyperpigmentation by inhibiting melanin synthesis. Glutathione, a powerful antioxidant, can also help lighten hyperpigmented areas and even out skin tone. Niacinamide, a form of vitamin B3, helps regulate melanin production and can fade dark spots and pigmentation irregularities.

Sensitive Skin

Sensitive skin is prone to irritation, redness, and reactivity. Probiotic supplements contain beneficial bacteria that promote a healthy gut microbiome, which in turn can improve skin health. Probiotics can help reduce skin inflammation and strengthen the skin barrier. Omega-3 fatty acids provide anti-inflammatory benefits, helping to soothe sensitive skin and reduce redness. Vitamin E, a potent antioxidant, protects the skin from environmental aggressors and helps calm and nourish sensitive skin.

Understanding Supplement Labels and Dosages

Reading Supplement Labels: Key Ingredients and Potency

When selecting skin supplements, it's essential to carefully read and understand the information provided on the product labels. Pay attention to the list of key ingredients and their respective quantities or potencies. Look for supplements that clearly state the specific nutrients or compounds they contain, such as vitamins, minerals, antioxidants, or herbal extracts.

Additionally, check for any additional ingredients or fillers that may be included in the supplement. Some individuals may have sensitivities or allergies to certain substances, so it's crucial to be aware of the complete ingredient list.

Recommended Dosages: Understanding the Optimal Intake

Dosages of supplements can vary depending on the specific nutrient and the desired effect. It's important to follow the recommended dosage guidelines provided on the product packaging or consult with a healthcare professional to determine the optimal intake for your needs.

Keep in mind that exceeding the recommended dosage does not necessarily result in better outcomes. In fact, taking excessive amounts of certain nutrients can be harmful. Stick to the recommended dosages unless otherwise advised by a healthcare professional.

Choosing Reliable Brands

When it comes to supplements, quality and safety are paramount. Choose supplements from reputable and reliable brands that follow Good Manufacturing Practices (GMP) and undergo third-party testing for quality and purity.

Look for certifications or seals of approval from independent organizations, such as the United States Pharmacopeia (USP) or ConsumerLab, which test and verify the quality of supplements. These certifications provide assurance that the product meets certain standards of safety and effectiveness.

Incorporating Supplements into Your Skincare Routine: Consulting with a Dermatologist!

Before adding any new supplements to your skincare routine, it's highly recommended to consult with a healthcare professional, such as a dermatologist or nutritionist. They can assess your specific skin concerns, overall health, and medication history to provide personalized recommendations.

A healthcare professional can help determine which supplements are most suitable for your needs and guide you on the appropriate dosages. They can also address any questions or concerns you may have and monitor your progress over time.

Potential Interactions with Medications

It's important to be aware of potential interactions between supplements and medications you may be taking. Some supplements can interfere with the absorption or effectiveness of certain medications, while others may enhance their effects.

Inform your healthcare professional about all medications, including over-the-counter drugs and herbal supplements, that you are currently taking. They can advise on any precautions or adjustments that may be necessary to ensure the safety and effectiveness of both your medication and supplement regimens.

Finding the Right Formulation

Skin supplements come in various formulations, including pills, capsules, powders, and liquids. Consider your personal preferences and lifestyle when choosing the right formulation for you.

Pills and capsules are convenient and easy to incorporate into your daily routine. Powders can be mixed with water or added to smoothies, providing flexibility in dosage and customization. Liquids can be consumed directly or added to beverages, offering quick absorption.

Remember to follow the recommended instructions for each formulation, including proper storage and handling.

Timing and Consistency

To maximize the benefits of skin supplements, it's important to establish a consistent routine. Take your supplements at the same time each day to help maintain steady levels of nutrients in your body.

Some supplements may be recommended to be taken with food, while others are best taken on an empty stomach. Follow the instructions provided by the manufacturer or consult with your healthcare professional for specific guidance.

Potential Risks and Side Effects of Skin Supplements

Allergic Reactions and Sensitivities

While skin supplements are generally safe for most individuals, there is a possibility of experiencing allergic reactions or sensitivities to certain ingredients. Some people may have specific allergies to substances commonly found in supplements, such as shellfish-derived glucosamine or certain herbal extracts.

If you have a known allergy or sensitivity to any ingredients, it's important to carefully read the labels and avoid supplements that contain those substances. Additionally, if you experience any signs of an allergic reaction, such as itching, rash, swelling, or difficulty breathing, discontinue use immediately and seek medical attention.

Overdosing and Toxicity

Taking excessive amounts of certain supplements can lead to overdosing and potential toxicity. This is especially true for fat-soluble vitamins, such as vitamin A and vitamin E, which can accumulate in the body over time.

It's crucial to follow the recommended dosage guidelines provided on the supplement packaging or as advised by a healthcare professional.

Taking more than the recommended amount does not necessarily result in better outcomes and can have adverse effects on your health.

If you are taking other medications or supplements, be cautious of potential interactions that may increase the risk of toxicity. Some nutrients, such as zinc or iron, can interfere with the absorption of other medications when taken in high doses. Always consult with a healthcare professional before starting any new supplement regimen, especially if you have underlying health conditions or are currently taking medications. They can provide personalized guidance and help you determine the appropriate dosages to minimize the risk of overdosing or toxicity.

While oral skin supplements can be a useful tool for improving skin health and reducing the signs of aging, it is important to remember that they are not a magic solution. It is essential to maintain a healthy diet and lifestyle, get plenty of sleep, and protect the skin from the sun and other environmental factors to achieve the best possible results.

SECTION ELEVEN

Travel and Skin Care

SECTION ELEVEN

Travel and Skin Care

Explore, Protect, and Glow!

Traveling can be an exciting and enriching experience, but it can also disrupt our skincare routine. Changes in climate, exposure to different environments, and the stress of travel can take a toll on our skin. In this section, we will delve into practical tips and strategies to help you maintain healthy skin while on the go, ensuring that your skin stays radiant and nourished throughout your journey.

Preparing Your Skin Before You Go

- **Assess Your Skincare Needs:** Consider the climate and conditions of your travel destination. Will you be exposed to extreme heat, dryness, or humidity? Adjust your skincare routine and product selection accordingly to address specific concerns. For example, if you're heading to a sunny beach destination, prioritize sun protection and hydration.

- **Pack Travel-Sized Essentials:** To save space and comply with airline regulations, opt for travel-sized skincare products. Transfer your favorite products into travel-friendly containers or invest in pre-packaged travel kits available from many skincare brands. Include essentials such as a gentle cleanser, moisturizer, sunscreen, and any targeted treatments you regularly use.

- **Sun Protection:** Regardless of your destination, sun protection is essential. Pack a broad-spectrum sunscreen with a high SPF and choose a travel-friendly option like a roll-on or a compact-sized sunscreen stick for easy application. Remember to apply sunscreen generously and reapply every two hours, especially if you'll be spending a lot of time outdoors.

Simplify Your Routine

a. **Streamline Your Skincare:** Traveling often means limited time and resources for an elaborate skincare routine. Simplify your routine to the essentials – a gentle cleanser, moisturizer, and sunscreen. Consider multi-purpose products like tinted moisturizers or lip balms with SPF to save time and space without compromising skincare effectiveness.

b. **Opt for Dual-Purpose Products:** Look for skincare products that offer multiple benefits. For example, a moisturizer with built-in antioxidants can provide hydration and protect against environmental stressors. This reduces the number of products you need to carry while ensuring your skin receives the necessary nourishment and protection.

Hydration is Key

a. **Drink Water:** Staying hydrated is crucial for your overall health and skin condition. Carry a reusable water bottle and drink plenty of water throughout your journey to maintain optimal hydration levels. If you're traveling to a destination with limited access to clean water, consider carrying a portable water purifier.

b. **Facial Mists and Hydrating Masks:** Refresh your skin during long flights or in dry environments with a hydrating facial mist. Look for mists that contain soothing ingredients like aloe vera or rosewater to combat dryness and rejuvenate your skin.

Additionally, consider using a hydrating sheet mask or overnight mask to provide intense hydration and restore moisture to your skin.

Protect and Cleanse

a. **Cleanse Regularly:** Traveling exposes your skin to pollution, sweat, and environmental impurities. Cleanse your face in the morning and evening to remove dirt and excess oil. Consider using a gentle, travel-friendly cleanser that won't strip your skin of its natural oils. If you prefer double cleansing, use a gentle oil-based cleanser followed by a water-based cleanser.

b. **Don't Forget Makeup Removal:** Removing makeup is crucial to prevent clogged pores and breakouts. Carry makeup remover wipes or travel-sized micellar water for easy and effective makeup removal on the go. Follow up with a gentle cleanser to ensure your skin is thoroughly clean before applying any skincare products.

Adjust to Climate

a. **Moisturize Accordingly:** Different climates can affect your skin's hydration needs. In dry climates, use a richer moisturizer to prevent moisture loss and keep your skin hydrated throughout the day. Look for moisturizers with ingredients like hyaluronic acid or ceramides to provide long-lasting hydration. In humid environments, opt for a lightweight, oil-free moisturizer to avoid feeling greasy while still maintaining hydration. Consider carrying a travel-sized facial mist to refresh and hydrate your skin throughout the day.

b. **Humidify:** If you're traveling to a dry destination or spending a lot of time in air-conditioned environments, consider using a portable humidifier in your hotel room to combat dryness and maintain skin hydration. A humidifier adds moisture to the air, which can help prevent your skin from becoming dry and flaky.

c. **Climate-Specific Skincare:** Depending on your destination, you may need to adjust your skincare routine to address specific climate-related concerns. For example, if you're traveling to a cold climate, incorporate a richer moisturizer and lip balm to protect your skin from harsh winds and low temperatures. In hot and humid climates, opt for lightweight, oil-free products that won't clog pores and contribute to breakouts.

Protect Your Skin from Environmental Factors

a. **Shield from the Sun:** Besides sunscreen, consider additional ways to protect your skin from the sun's harmful rays. Wear wide-brimmed hats, sunglasses, and lightweight, breathable clothing that covers exposed skin. Seek shade during peak sun hours, typically between ten a.m. and four p.m.

b. **Minimize Airplane Cabin Effects:** Airplane cabins can be dehydrating due to low humidity levels. Combat dryness by applying a hydrating moisturizer before and during the flight. Drink plenty of water, and avoid alcohol and caffeine, as they can further dehydrate your skin.

c. **Combat Pollution:** If you're traveling to a highly polluted area, take extra measures to protect your skin. Use antioxidant-rich skincare products to combat free radicals caused by pollution.

Maintain a Healthy Lifestyle

a. **Balanced Diet:** Nourish your skin from within by maintaining a balanced diet. Consume fruits, vegetables, and foods rich in antioxidants to support healthy skin. Avoid excessive consumption of processed foods and sugary snacks, as they can contribute to inflammation and breakouts.

b. **Get Enough Sleep:** Traveling can disrupt your sleep schedule, but try to prioritize restful sleep. Lack of sleep can affect your skin's appearance and make it look dull and tired. Create a relaxing bedtime routine and ensure you're getting enough rest to allow your skin to rejuvenate.

c. **Reduce Stress:** Traveling can be stressful, but excessive stress can impact your skin's health. Practice stress management techniques like deep breathing exercises, meditation, or engaging in activities that bring you joy. Stress reduction promotes a healthy complexion.

Maintaining healthy skin while traveling requires a proactive approach and adjustments to your skincare routine. By preparing your skin before you go, simplifying your routine, staying hydrated, protecting and cleansing your skin, adjusting to different climates, and practicing a healthy lifestyle, you can ensure that your skin remains nourished and radiant throughout your journey. Remember, taking care of your skin goes beyond the destination—it's a lifelong commitment. So, embrace your travel adventures while prioritizing the well-being of your skin. Safe travels!

Embrace Your Skin's Radiance

As we reach the end of this skincare journey together, remember that true beauty begins with self-care and self-love. Your skin is unique, just like you, and it deserves to be nurtured and celebrated. Armed with the knowledge gained from this book, you are now equipped to make informed decisions about your skincare routine.

But skincare is more than just following a regimen—it's about embracing your skin's natural radiance; it's about accepting and loving yourself, flaws and all. Remember that true beauty is not solely determined by external appearances but by the confidence and authenticity that shine from within.

As you embark on your skincare adventure, let curiosity be your guide. Continue to explore new ingredients, techniques, and trends, but always listen to your skin and honor its needs. Treat yourself to moments of self-care, finding joy in the rituals that nourish both your skin and your soul.

And never forget the power of consistency. Skincare is a journey, not a destination. Embrace the daily commitment to caring for your skin, knowing that each small action adds up to long-term results. Celebrate the progress you make, even on days when the mirror may not reflect the changes you desire.

Finally, share your newfound knowledge and passion with others. Be a source of inspiration and encouragement, reminding those around you of the importance of self-care and self-love. Together, we can create a world where skincare is not just a beauty routine, but a transformative act of self-empowerment.

As you close this book, remember that your skin is unique, and your journey is your own. Embrace it, celebrate it, and let your skin's natural radiance shine through. You have the power to unlock your best skin and reveal your most beautiful self.

If you want to, you can reach out to us at: www.goodskinbadskin.com or www.dermosphere.com

You can also email us at: dermosphere@gmail.com

Here's to a lifetime of radiant, healthy, and confident skin!